LIVING WELL WITH EPILEPSY

D0947359

Living Well with Epilepsy

Robert J. Gumnit, M.D.

Director, MINCEP Epilepsy Care, P.A.
and
Clinical Professor of Neurology and Neurosurgery
University of Minnesota
Minneapolis, Minnesota

$\mathcal{D}$*emos*

WESTERN IOWA TECH - LIBRARY
22369

Demos Publications, 156 Fifth Avenue, New York, New York 10010

© 1990 by Demos Publications, Inc. All rights reserved. This book is protected by copyright. No part of it may be reproduced, stored in a retrieval
system, or transmitted in any form or by any means, electronic, mechanical,
photocopying, recording, or otherwise, without the prior written permission
of the publisher.

Made in the United States of America

Great care has been taken to maintain the accuracy of the information contained in this volume. However, neither the author nor Demos Publications
can be held responsible for errors or for any consequences arising from the
use of the information contained herein.

ISBN: 0-939957-24-8
ISBN: 0-939957-21-3 (paperback)
LC: 89-85237

PREFACE

Epilepsy is a disorder in which the patient may be impaired for only a few minutes a week, but may otherwise be totally disabled. While proper medical treatment is essential to bring seizures under control, much more can and should be done to minimize the disability associated with epilepsy and maximize the satisfactions of life.

There *are* realistic limitations introduced by uncontrolled seizures and the side-effects of antiepileptic drugs. The real issue for most patients, however, is their place in society: how they view themselves, how they are viewed by others, and the changes in normal everyday life that epilepsy introduces.

To live successfully with a chronic medical problem requires extra thought, good planning, and realistic self-assessment.

There are people with mistaken ideas who behave thoughtlessly and prejudicially toward others, especially those who are handicapped, although, for the most part, people are taken at their own evaluation. If you present yourself as competent and responsible, you will be treated that way. There is a powerful lesson to be learned. There are enough real limitations placed on people in this world as it is. We don't have to introduce unnecessary ones.

This book is designed to give people with seizures, and others who share the adventure of life with them, the information and the outlook necessary to live successfully with epilepsy. They need to take charge of their lives and to venture boldly into new experiences. It is not the limitations that life has placed on them but the strengths and resources that they possess that determine who they are and what they will become.

This book is the distillation of 30 years of experience in treating people with epilepsy. In particular, the past 15 years at MINCEP have taught the authors about the varieties of experiences and the broad repertoire of responses that people with epilepsy can have. Hopefully, the approach presented in this book to the multi-faceted problems facing a person with epilepsy will provide stimulation to other health-care providers. The book should be particularly useful to physicians, nurses, psychologists, social workers, EEG technologists, physical and occupational therapists, teachers, vocational rehabilitation counselors, and others who help people with epilepsy everywhere.

Robert J. Gumnit

ACKNOWLEDGMENTS

This book would not have been possible without the skilled professional help of Michael P. Moore. His ability to put our thoughts into a useful form was invaluable.

Sophie Reuben, MSW, played a major role in shaping my own and MINCEP's approach to the patient with epilepsy. Her skill in getting to the heart of the matter, in casting off the irrelevant, and helping focus action where it is meaningful has been exemplary.

In a similar manner, Florence Gray played an important role, not only in stimulating the writing of this book, but in focusing our energies. All of the contributors owe an enormous debt to our patients and our co-workers at Abbott-Northwestern Hospital, the Gillette Children's Hospital, and the University of Minnesota Hospitals who have taught us so much.

CONTENTS

CONTRIBUTORS

Richard V. Andrews, M.D., Pediatric Neurologist, MINCEP Epilepsy Care, P.A., and Clinical Instructor, University of Minnesota, Minneapolis.

Judy L. Antonello, A.C.S.W., L.I.C.S.W., Clinical Social Worker, MINCEP Epilepsy Care, P.A., Minneapolis.

Lisa M. Butler, R.N., Pediatric Nurse Clinician, MINCEP Epilepsy Care, P.A., Minneapolis.

Connie Frazer, R.N., Nurse Clinician, MINCEP Epilepsy Care, P.A., Minneapolis.

John R. Gates, M.D., Medical Director, MINCEP Epilepsy Care, P.A., and Clinical Associate Professor of Neurology and Neurosurgery, University of Minnesota, Minneapolis.

Florence Gray, Associate Director, Epilepsy Research Center, University of Minnesota, Minneapolis.

Robert J. Gumnit, M.D., Director, MINCEP Epilepsy Care, P.A., and Clinical Professor of Neurology and Neurosurgery, University of Minnesota, Minneapolis.

Douglas G. Heck, Ph.D., Clinical Psychologist, MINCEP Epilepsy Care, P.A., Minneapolis.

Ilo E. Leppik, M.D., Director of Pharmacologic Research, MINCEP Epilepsy Care, P.A., and Clinical Professor of Neurology and Pharmacy, University of Minnesota, Minneapolis.

Robert E. Maxwell, M.D., Ph.D., F.A.C.S., Associate Professor of Neurosurgery, University of Minnesota, Minneapolis.

Frank J. Ritter, M.D., Pediatric Neurologist, MINCEP Epilepsy Care, P.A., and Clinical Instructor, University of Minnesota, Minneapolis.

Tess Sierzant, R.N., B.S.N., Nurse Clinician, MINCEP Epilepsy Care, P.A., Minneapolis.

Mark S. Yerby, M.D., M.P.H., Neurologist, MINCEP Epilepsy Care, P.A., and Clinical Associate Professor, University of Minnesota, Minneapolis.

Living Successfully with Epilepsy

Robert J. Gumnit, M.D.

Congratulations! The fact that you are reading this book indicates that you have made a decision to take control of your epilepsy. Or you may have decided to help a child or other loved one take control. Following up on that decision by seeking more information is probably the most important step you can take.

This book provides the latest information about epilepsy, but it will also give you much more. The authors are health professionals with many years of experience helping people with epilepsy take charge and live normal and productive lives. Our patients have taught us how epilepsy can be made a part of a very fulfilling life.

We at MINCEP Epilepsy Care—"Minnesota's Comprehensive Epilepsy Program"—have learned that it is not the severity of a person's epilepsy that has the greatest effect on how well he or she will live. Most patients who do well do so because they have learned to cope with their epilepsy. They find out how it is possible to do what they want to do in life, and then do it. Two people can have the same level of seizure activity, but one lives a depressed, inactive life, the other a happy, fulfilling one. The difference is the result of their mental attitude.

Of course, life with epilepsy may not be easy. Some occupations, such as law enforcement and the military, do not accept people with epilepsy. In addition, depending on how well controlled his seizures are, an individual may have to accept certain limitations. But people who take charge of their lives and who are assertive about getting help when needed and doing things for themselves whenever possible can and will lead happy and fulfilling lives.

GETTING STARTED

If you or a loved one has just been diagnosed as having epilepsy, you are probably experiencing a swirling of emotions within you. Fear, anger, worry, sadness, helplessness, guilt; these and many other feelings are all perfectly understandable and normal. Experiencing them is part of the process of accepting epilepsy and beginning to cope with it. You must deal with each emotion, face the fact of epilepsy, find out that there is nothing you could have done to prevent it, and know that you can learn to cope with it and minimize its negative impact on your life.

The first time you heard that you or a loved one had epilepsy, that is probably all you heard. Any other information about the disorder and any medications that may have been prescribed were probably forgotten in the emotional turmoil of the moment. That too is normal; you should feel comfortable about scheduling another appointment to go over that information again and to discuss how you are feeling.

In fact, this is the perfect time to start practicing being assertive in your relationship with your doctor and the other people taking care of your family. Write down questions as you think of them, and bring them to each visit. Tell them what you need and how you feel, listen to them, and continue to ask for explanations until you are satisfied. Chapter 5 has more suggestions on working with your health-care team.

Most people think that epilepsy is a disease that causes seizures. That is not quite true, since epilepsy is not a disease as such. There are hundreds of causes of seizures, ranging from head injuries to meningitis. Making a diagnosis of epilepsy means only that a person has had more than one seizure. The doctor must still try to find their cause. Unfortunately, sometimes no specific cause can be identified.

Having a seizure does not mean that a person is "going crazy" or has some terrible brain disease. It does not mean that his brain is starting to rot or that he is retarded. Epilepsy is not communicable—it cannot spread from one person to another. These ideas may seem bizarre, but all have been expressed by people who thought they knew about epilepsy.

What is a seizure? A seizure is simply a symptom of some temporary disturbance of brain activity. In fact, everyone is capable of having a seizure. For example, if an airplane flying at a high altitude were to suddenly lose its air pressure, the loss of oxygen would cause everyone aboard to have a seizure. Not everyone on that airplane would have a seizure at the same time, however. This is because each person may have a different *threshold* for seizures—the level at which seizures will occur. Some people have a higher threshold than others and may never experience a seizure. Others have a low threshold and may have recurring seizures; they have epilepsy. *More than two million people (about 1% of the population) in the United States have epilepsy.*

The fact that a seizure threshold exists for everyone is very important in controlling epilepsy. Certain medications can be taken regularly to keep an individual's threshold above the point at which his seizures occur. By finding out what type of brain activity is present during a patient's seizure, what that person is doing when the seizure occurs, and how the seizure affects his body, a specialist in treating epilepsy—a neurologist—can decide what treatment is appropriate. The aim of therapy is to prevent more seizures. Even one or two seizures a year is too many, because of the danger of injury and the social problems that may result from them.

Keeping track of all the necessary information is where the patient and family play a major role. It is very important to tell your neurologist everything you can remember about when the first seizure occurred. This will help the physician in deciding which medication to prescribe to try to prevent a second seizure.

There are two things family members must do in case a second seizure occurs. The first is to learn some simple first aid steps (see Chapter 9). The second is to keep a careful diary. Information on what type of seizure occurs, when it occurs, and when medication is taken will help the neurologist diagnose which type of seizure the person has, possible factors that caused the seizure, and what type of medication to give and in what dosage.

Other tests the neurologist can do to help decide how to treat a patient will be discussed in the next few chapters. What is very important at this point is to realize that *the patient and his or her family plays a major role in the treatment and control of epilepsy.* No matter how skilled the physicians and nurses are, epilepsy cannot be controlled without the patient and family working together with their health-care team.

How Do I Feel About Having Epilepsy?

Some people with chronic disorders, such as diabetes, arthritis, or epilepsy, dislike being called a diabetic, an arthritic, or an epileptic. We believe that those labels are derogatory only if the person with the disease lets them be. To the person with a good self-image, these are merely words that describe a certain factor in his or her life.

That is why it is very important to ask yourself how you feel about having epilepsy. Do you feel as if it has suddenly reared up and taken over your entire life? If so, it might be helpful to concentrate on all the good things you can do and set some good challenging goals for your future.

Seeing a family counselor shortly after epilepsy is diagnosed can be very helpful in sorting out all your feelings and those of your loved ones. If the person with epilepsy had a poor self-image before diagnosis, that self-image will probably become even worse unless help is sought. If the family was experiencing a stressful lifestyle or poor interpersonal relationships before diagnosis, epilepsy will add even more stress and divide the family still further.

Self-image and family relationships will be discussed in detail in later chapters, but they are mentioned here because poor adjustment to epilepsy and a poor self-image can get in the way of everything else the health-care team and individual can do. People with epilepsy must feel that they are worth taking care of, and the family must support them emotionally and in practical ways. Talking about feelings, making plans for the present and future, and setting goals are all powerful medicines for controlling epilepsy.

THE BASIS OF CONTROL

Doctors, nurses, the patient, and the family should be thought of as a *team*. Their job is to begin by obtaining a diagnosis, finding the right treatment, and then keeping the epilepsy well managed and under control. What will keep them traveling along the right track? Motivation!

Motivation is not just a reason for doing something, it is the power that gets things done. It starts with a strong self-image, a feeling that you deserve the best and have the ability to get it. Motivation is fostered by family members and friends willing to lend support and is guided by a personal achievement plan, which contains specific objectives you want to accomplish, what you will do to accomplish them, and how you will reward yourself when you accomplish each objective. The achievement plan is directed at a major goal in your life that you want to attain.

What is your goal? Is it to help a loved one control epilepsy, or to control your own epilepsy? If it is, that is understandable, but probably not the best goal in terms of providing motivation. Instead, try thinking of the specific steps in your treatment plan as your objectives and think of ways you can reward yourself or your loved one when the objectives are met each week, for example. Frequent simple rewards, like a movie, a ballgame, a meal at a restaurant, or simply praise for the person who succeeded in meeting his objectives, will provide a solid basis for success.

With the epilepsy under good control thanks to achieving the treatment objectives, you can then decide what your next goal will be. What is your purpose in life? What really gets you excited? Is it having a family, or being a scientist, or learning to dance, or earning a place on an athletic team, or earning a college degree, or opening up your own business? Whatever it is, write it down and describe it as clearly and enthusiastically as you can, and then work out the steps you will take to make it happen.

Whenever you feel low on motivation, or perhaps that controlling epilepsy is not that important, refer to your achievement plan. Getting excited about meeting your objectives and achieving your goal will be the fuel you need to keep going. Setbacks will occur, as they do to everyone, but by understanding what motivates you and going right back to doing the things you know will help you succeed, you will be a successful, productive, enthusiastic person, who just happens to have epilepsy.

THE WHO'S WHO OF EPILEPSY

Epilepsy has been recognized throughout history. The word comes from the ancient Greek word "epilepsia," which means seizure. It was a sacred disease in ancient Egypt because of the belief that a god had entered the person. In medieval times, epilepsy was called the "falling sickness" and was thought to be caused by demons possessing the person.

Many notable figures in history have had epilepsy: Socrates, Alexander the Great, Julius Caesar, Alfred Nobel, and Thomas Edison. Today there are people with epilepsy represented among the writers, artists, scientists, politicians, and sports stars of the world.

Does this mean that epilepsy gives a person certain special powers? Well, yes and no. It does affect the brain, but there is no evidence to support the idea that it increases a person's intelligence or creative abilities. There is one way that epilepsy can help to make a person successful, though. Like all other chronic conditions, epilepsy forces an individual to focus on what is important in life. It requires constant attention to a treatment plan, which, if followed, teaches the person to control his or her own life. Epilepsy can even make a person stronger because of the challenge it presents. The same skills built by controlling epilepsy will be valuable assets when it comes to accomplishing other goals in life.

Epilepsy is a challenge. The rest of this book will help you learn and think about the things you can do to meet that challenge. Keep reminding yourself why you are reading this book and apply what you learn. Remember your motivation in life!

2

Understanding Epilepsy

Robert J. Gumnit, M.D.

A diagnosis of epilepsy usually unleashes a torrent of questions from the patient and family: Why do the seizures happen? What could I have done to prevent them? Will I be able to prevent any more seizures from occurring? If they do occur, will they get any better or worse? Can epilepsy be cured, or will I have it for the rest of my life?

Sometimes people feel guilty, thinking that in some way they caused the seizures or failed to prevent them. Sometimes they are angry that epilepsy happened to them or a loved one.

The answers to all these questions are different for each patient. Often there are no firm answers, just educated guesses by the doctor. The family can be reassured that there was nothing they could have done to prevent the seizures from occurring in the first place. They can also be reassured that most people with epilepsy achieve very good control of their seizures, meaning they occur rarely if ever. And sometimes epilepsy can indeed be cured through special surgery. There is a good deal of hope that even more people will be helped in the near future, as medical researchers discover new drugs to prevent seizures and develop new techniques for eliminating their causes.

It is important that you ask all the questions you have about seizures and epilepsy, because information will be your best tool against the disorder. Correct information will also dispel unfounded fears that many people have about epilepsy (Am I going crazy?). Don't be afraid that you won't be able to understand or remember everything you are told. No one can absorb all this information at once, especially while still reeling from the shock of diagnosis. Take some time to examine your feelings about epilepsy, and write down your questions and things you want to discuss.

This chapter will explain what a seizure is and discuss the different kinds of seizures that can occur. It will also explain what is known about the causes of various types of epilepsy. This information will help you understand more about the type of epilepsy you or your loved one has. Most importantly, it will help you to become more involved in treating the epilepsy and, if possible, preventing future seizures.

WHAT IS A SEIZURE?

Surprisingly, few people with epilepsy ask what a seizure actually is. Everything they know about what happens to them during a seizure is based on what they have been told by family members and friends who have witnessed their seizures. But more people should ask what happens inside them during a seizure, or what it really means when a person has epilepsy. A better understanding of seizures and the different types of epilepsy will help you become actively involved in treating your epilepsy.

Seizures can be divided into two general categories: epileptic seizures and nonepileptic seizures. An *epileptic seizure* is an episode of disturbed brain activity that results in abnormal behavior. The main problem lies in the brain. A *nonepileptic seizure* is an episode of abnormal behavior that is not caused mainly by a disturbance in brain activity, but by some other problem. Abrupt drops in blood pressure, an imbalance of body fluids or chemicals, or certain psychological problems can cause nonepileptic seizures.

Several tests can be done to determine whether a person has epileptic or nonepileptic seizures (some people have both). They include blood and urine tests, neurological examinations that show how a person's brain is controlling muscle and nerve responses, EEG (electroencephalography), which monitors brain activity, and various types of radiological studies and brain scans that produce pictures of the brain and show how it is working. These tests will be described in detail in Chapter 6.

Epileptic seizures are caused by sudden, uncontrolled bursts of electrical activity from brain cells. Because the brain controls all behavior, an epileptic seizure causes a person to behave in an unusual way. Some people can feel a seizure coming on through a sensation known as an *aura*. This sensation is actually a minor seizure caused by abnormal activity in one part of the brain. The warning is usually the same every time an individual has a seizure, but each person will experience a different aura. For some people, the aura will be all there is to the seizure, while others will have a seizure with no warning aura. Feelings before, during, and after seizures will be discussed in greater detail in Chapter 6.

A seizure may result in many different behavioral changes. The person may be unable to focus attention and may stare blankly, not responding to other people. Or, the person may lose control of muscles or have a muscle spasm, or may have convulsions (rhythmic, uncontrolled shaking of a body part or the whole body). The person may lose bladder control, wetting his or her clothes. Many people lose consciousness during a seizure.

Most epileptic seizures are brief, lasting less than two minutes. When the seizure is over and the person regains awareness or consciousness, she may be panicky and confused, have difficulty speaking, have a headache, have weakness in some part of the body, and may be very tired. Most people don't remember what happened just before and during the seizure.

IS EPILEPSY A DISEASE?

Epilepsy should not really be described as a disease because recurrent seizures can be caused by many very different diseases. The term epilepsy refers to a chronic (lasting a long time) disorder in which the individual either has recurrent seizures caused by disturbances in brain activity, or would have such seizures if not controlled by medications.

We would not say that a person had epilepsy if, for example, two or three seizures occurred during an illness such as meningitis, but stopped after the illness was treated. But we would make the diagnosis of epilepsy if a person had two seizures weeks or months apart. In other words, a seizure is a symptom of a problem that is causing a disturbance in the brain. If doctors can't find a short-term cause for the seizure and the person goes on to have more, then doctors would say that the patient has the disorder called epilepsy.

When someone first has a seizure, it is very important to see a doctor to try to determine what caused the seizure. The doctor will take a complete history of the person's health and the health of family members. He will also need as much of a description of the seizure as possible to help in making a diagnosis. Treatment will depend, of course, on whether the doctor determines that the patient has had an epileptic or nonepileptic seizure.

To say that someone has epilepsy means only that the person has recurrent seizures. A more complete description of his disorder would include the type of epilepsy he has, and the kind of seizures he experiences.

WHAT ARE THE DIFFERENT TYPES OF EPILEPSY?

Epilepsy is classified by the specialists in this area into three major divisions. In *partial (focal)* epilepsy, the seizures are focused in a limited portion of the brain. In *generalized* epilepsy either no specific part of the brain can be identified as the source of the seizures or the part that starts the seizure causes the whole brain to become involved. In epilepsy of *unknown etiology* (origin), monitoring has been unable to detect abnormal brain activity or has produced unclear results.

Other information, such as age, a family history of epilepsy if any, how epilepsy developed, and the kinds of seizures experienced, are additional factors in classifying epilepsy. Each of these broad categories can be subdivided into different epileptic syndromes.

WHAT ARE THE DIFFERENT KINDS OF SEIZURES?

Seizures are described, or classified, by the behavior and EEG changes that occur *during the seizure.* The following descriptions are simplified from the seizure classifications established by physicians who specialize in treating and studying epilepsy.

1. Partial seizures, which begin in one part of the brain, can be classified as simple partial, complex partial, or tonic–clonic. *Simple partial seizures* cause one kind of movement or a strange sensation such as emotion, smell, taste, or dizziness. In *complex partial seizures,* the person loses awareness as the seizure begins or loses awareness after having a simple partial seizure. Almost two-thirds of people with epilepsy have complex partial seizures. Partial seizures that proceed (secondarily generalize) to what are called *tonic–clonic convulsions* cause the body to become rigid (tonic), usually causing the person to fall to the ground and then to begin shaking or jerking as the muscles relax rhythmically (clonic).
2. Generalized seizures affect the whole body at the start of the seizure. This type of seizure causes a loss of consciousness. Generalized seizures are characterized by impaired consciousness affecting the whole body. The person may have an *absence seizure,* in which awareness of surroundings is cut off; jerking of whole muscle groups (*clonic seizures*); muscle rigidity (*tonic seizure*); a *tonic–clonic seizure,* in which the person's body becomes stiff (tonic phase), he falls, followed by alternating stiffening and relaxation (clonic phase); or an *atonic seizure,* in which all the muscles suddenly relax, causing a collapse and fall.
3. *Unclassified seizure* is the last category, so named because not enough information is available about the person's seizures.

A person with epilepsy may only experience one kind of seizure or several different kinds, either during the same episode or at different times. Every effort must be made by the doctor, family, and person with epilepsy to determine what kinds of seizures the person has. This information is crucial to achieving the best treatment for the seizures.

Psychogenic Seizures

Some individuals experience seizures that appear to be caused by disturbances in brain activity but are really not. Some people think they have experienced a seizure but are actually misinterpreting a sensory experience or temporary feeling such as dizziness, inability to concentrate, or forgetfulness. Others experience true episodes of abnormal behavior that appear to be seizures, but when monitored by an EEG, show no brain disturbance. These episodes of nonepileptic seizures appear to be caused by psychological stress, misinterpretation, or other mental factors. They are called *psychogenic seizures,* a term that reflects their psychological cause.

Some people may experience some psychogenic seizures as well as seizures that are caused by epilepsy. These people need to take antiepileptic medications, but they may also need counseling to find the cause of the psychogenic seizures. People who have only psychogenic seizures are not helped by the medications prescribed for epilepsy. In fact, they may be made worse if the drugs are given in high doses in an attempt to stop the seizures. For this reason, and to help find the psychological cause of the person's seizures, it is necessary to study the person closely to try to determine if he or she is having psychogenic seizures or epileptic seizures, or perhaps both.

If it is clear that someone is having psychogenic seizures, professional counseling can help find the cause and treat the emotional problem.

BEGINNING TO COPE WITH EPILEPSY

Because they involve loss of control, epileptic seizures are dangerous, and they can be embarrassing. The person with epilepsy may feel ashamed or angry. Children or unthinking adults may add to the problem, ridiculing the individual or making too much of a fuss about the seizure. This is indeed unfortunate, but public education is helping people understand—rather than fear—epilepsy.

The person with epilepsy, family, and friends can help by learning and teaching the public simple first-aid steps to take when someone has a seizure (see Chapter 9). They can also help by not hiding their epilepsy. Talking openly and honestly about what it is and how it affects their lives helps. This is certainly not easy, but it is actually much easier and more productive than hiding the disorder and fearing the inevitable discovery.

As you begin to understand and accept epilepsy, you will become better able to become actively involved in its treatment. This treatment should begin as soon as a diagnosis is made. Its aim is to control seizures completely. The next chapter will describe what is known about the causes of epilepsy and how the disorder is treated.

3

The Causes and Treatment of Epilepsy

Robert J. Gumnit, M.D.

Epilepsy can rarely be cured. Therefore, the goal of treatment is to control the seizures, so that they will occur rarely, if ever. However, the treatment must not cause other health problems or prevent normal functioning. Developing a treatment plan that can balance these factors and result in the highest possible quality of life requires a team effort in which the patient and family are the most important members.

One of the first challenges for the team is to try to determine what has caused the epileptic seizures. There are many possible causes of epilepsy, but in about half the cases no specific cause can be positively identified. If a cause can be found, that information can be very helpful in deciding how to treat the epilepsy.

This chapter focuses on what is known about the causes of epilepsy and discusses what options are available to the individual and doctor in treating those causes. Later, in Chapter 6, the various procedures and tests that can be used to diagnose epilepsy and identify kinds of seizures will be described.

WHAT CAUSES EPILEPSY?

The known causes of epilepsy are as follows.

1. Inherited diseases such as phenylketonuria (PKU), tuberous sclerosis, and neurofibromatosis can cause a person to have recurrent seizures.
2. An inherited tendency to develop epilepsy. About 2% of the general population develops epilepsy by age 40. When one parent or a brother or sister has epilepsy, there is about a 5% chance that a child will develop epilepsy. This is because the child may inherit a lower than normal seizure threshold or level of stimulus at which a seizure is triggered. The inherited tendency is more likely to cause epilepsy to develop in childhood than later in life. You may wish to consult a

11

genetic counselor for more specific information about your family's situation.

3. Problems occurring during the development of a fetus, which can be caused by such things as the mother being exposed to certain medications, street drugs, alcohol, infections, or injury.
4. Problems occurring during birth, such as lack of oxygen, damage from forceps delivery, or other injury to the baby's brain.
5. Head injuries at any time of life that are severe enough to cause an injury to the brain. A seizure may occur at the time of a head injury or even two or three years later, but the person does not have epilepsy unless repeated seizures occur at different times.
6. A tumor (abnormal growth of tissue) in the brain.
7. A blood clot or abnormal blood vessel formation in the brain.

TREAT THE CAUSE OR TREAT THE SEIZURES?

Some of the more specific causes above, such as a brain tumor or blood clot, can be treated directly. In these cases, the strategy is to treat the *cause* of the epilepsy to try to prevent the person's seizures.

When epilepsy has a more general cause, such as an inherited tendency to have seizures or a head injury that causes repeated seizures, the strategy will be to find a treatment that prevents the seizures. The same strategy will apply if no specific cause can be identified. If your doctor has identified a cause, try to accept that information as a positive step toward finding the best possible treatment. Remember that no one is to blame for the kinds of things that usually cause epilepsy, such as inheritance, an unavoidable accident, or a brain tumor. Remember, in most cases, no definite cause can be found.

And if epilepsy has resulted from an accident caused by negligence, it is important to separate the process of resolving that problem from the challenge of controlling epilepsy. This can be very difficult to do, but it is a crucial part of developing a positive attitude, both for the family and for the individual with epilepsy. A professional counselor or social worker may prove very helpful at this time if you feel there are emotional or social problems that will stand in the way of controlling the epilepsy.

TREATMENT OF EPILEPSY

Medications

Epilepsy is most often treated with medications, which are referred to as *antiepileptic medications* or *anticonvulsants*. There are about 20 commonly used antiepileptic medications, but most people with epilepsy are successfully treated with one of three major types. These are described in Chapter 7.

Specific medications are prescribed to treat specific types of seizures. This means that if a person has more than one type of seizure, more than one drug may be prescribed. A combination of medications may also be prescribed if the person's seizures are difficult to control.

Finding the best medication, combination of medications, and dosage to control a person's seizures may take some time. The family and individual are crucial in this process. You must be sure you understand when to take the medication and do your best to follow the schedule as closely as possible. Be honest if you forget to take the medication and a seizure occurs. The situation will be made much worse if you deny the error, as the physician may erroneously conclude that the dosage is too low and increase it or that the medication is ineffective and suggest a change in drugs, unnecessarily. Also, if paying for the medication is a problem, don't be afraid to ask if a less-expensive brand is available, or if financial assistance is available.

Be sure to report any side-effects from the medication. Your doctor will tell you what to watch for. Write down and report immediately any unusual reactions you think might be caused by the medication. Fortunately, antiepileptic medications are generally safe, and serious side-effects are unusual. But because these medications act on the brain, they can cause drowsiness or confusion, especially if prescribed in large doses. Telling your doctor about these problems will allow you to work with him to achieve a treatment that both prevents seizures and allows mental alertness and physical energy.

Diet

A small number of children with certain types of seizures may be treated with a *ketogenic diet,* which includes a high intake of fats. It is not known how this diet helps prevent seizures. Diet is a very important part of treatment in people with *phenylketonuria,* or PKU. This disorder can be detected through newborn screening, and a special diet must be followed to help prevent health problems, including seizures.

Surgery

After extensive evaluation, some individuals with epilepsy may be candidates for brain surgery. Although uncommon, brain tumors are one cause of epilepsy in which surgery may be required.

Some people with uncontrolled partial or complex partial seizures may also be helped by surgery. These patients must meet two general qualifications: first, that their seizures have not been controlled by extensive attempts ·with antiepileptic medication therapy and, second, that their seizures can be traced to a certain small part of the brain, which will not cause major problems if removed. Some other patients who suffer from very severe generalized seizures that cause serious injury may also be helped by a type of brain surgery that attempts to reduce the severity of the seizures.

There have been major advances in brain surgery in recent years, but it is still a treatment that is suitable for only a small proportion of people with epilepsy. Even those who are helped by the removal of a small part of the brain usually continue to require medications to control seizures, Brain surgery is described in more detail in Chapter 8.

Uncontrolled Epilepsy

Sometimes medications are unable to control a person's seizures. Also, some individuals are unhappy with the quality of their lives, even though their seizures may be under control. These situations can usually be improved by taking a more aggressive approach toward diagnosis and treatment of seizures, and by paying attention to all parts of a person's lifestyle.

These improvements can best be made by working with a team of health professionals who are devoted to helping people with epilepsy live better lives. The next chapter describes how you can get this type of help if you so desire. It will also suggest ways to improve your working relationship with any health-care team you decide to see for epilepsy care.

4

Finding Your Way to High-Quality Care

Robert J. Gumnit, M.D.

We live in a time of rapidly improving health care, especially for people with chronic disorders such as epilepsy. Earlier in this century, physicians had all they could do to cope with infectious diseases—influenza, tuberculosis, and polio. People with chronic disorders either didn't live very long or were placed in institutions. There were no long-term effective treatments or drugs for most chronic disorders.

Today, there are effective treatments for many chronic health problems, including epilepsy. And there is also a new attitude—a team approach—directed at helping people live as well as possible with epilepsy. Doctors, nurses, and other health professionals know that positive results will come when a person and family are motivated to become involved in a team effort to deal with epilepsy.

That's good news—but only if you are able to gain access to care that will help you improve your life. Knowing how the health-care system works will help you find your way to a knowledgeable health-care team. Unfortunately, finding high-quality health care is not the only challenge. You also have to find a way to pay for it. Costs have increased dramatically, bringing changes in how health care is provided and how it is paid for. Some people with epilepsy, especially those without health insurance, find it difficult to get adequate health care. And even those who have health insurance need to know how to use it to their best advantage.

A key to obtaining the best possible control of epilepsy is being willing to search for—and fight for, if necessary—the highest-quality care. To succeed, you need to understand the health-care system and find a way to obtain and pay for the services you need. This chapter provides information and tips that will help you with this process.

CHANGES IN HEALTH CARE

It used to be fairly simple to obtain medical care. If you lived in a rural area, there was probably only one doctor to go to. If you lived in a city, you

15

chose a family doctor or generalist and went to him when you were sick. The doctor was essentially a private businessman; he sent you the bill, and you paid it as soon as you could. If you could not afford to pay, he sent you to a hospital or special medical center where charitable groups provided care to those who could not afford it.

We now live in a period of rapid change in the way health care is provided. Now, far fewer doctors work completely independently. Because of the higher cost of practicing medicine, most doctors are now partners in an office with others. These partners share the many costs of running a medical office, including rent, equipment, supplies, nurses, secretaries, receptionists, and billing. Many doctors work in clinics, where they are partners with a large group of other physicians, or they may work as employees of a large medical center. These changes mean that most physicians now have two responsibilities: to provide care to their patients, **and** to make sure the company or organization they are a part of makes a profit, or at least breaks even.

So, while we can be very grateful for the improvements that have occurred in health care, we also need to realize that it has become a huge business. In 1987, Americans spent more than $450 billion on health care. Most of this total was paid by patients themselves, partly through health insurance premiums. Part of it was paid by the public, through taxpayer support of federal Medicare for the elderly and Medicaid for the poor. However, an increasingly large part of the health-care bill was paid by employers who provide health insurance to their employees.

Many companies still provide the traditional type of health insurance—indemnity plans—that pays most or all of the medical expenses of an employee and family members and allows them to see any doctor they choose. But an increasing number of employers are signing contracts with a new type of medical service company called a "health maintenance organization," or HMO.

An HMO sells health services to employers, who in turn provide free or reduced-cost HMO memberships to their employees. HMO members are then entitled to go to those doctors who have signed contracts with the HMO, which pays them to provide specific health-care services agreed upon in the contract with the employer. The HMO will only pay part of the cost—and sometimes none of it—if the member goes to a doctor who does not have a contract with that HMO. Many HMOs also require members to see a general practitioner first, and only if he or she decides that the patient needs to see a specialist will the HMO pay for this type of care.

Some HMOs are more restrictive than others with respect to which doctors members can visit. One type, called a staff model HMO, or PPO, requires its members to visit special clinics run by its own employees and physicians. Most HMOs, however, sign contracts with doctors at many different types of clinics and offices.

HMOs are part of a large experiment in the way health care is provided and paid for in the United States. It is not clear if this restrictive service arrangement will answer the question: How can we as a nation afford to provide high-quality health care for everyone who needs it? While in some countries the government provides health insurance to all citizens, many fear that this would reduce the quality of care in the United States because of limited availability, increased bureaucracy, and decreased competition. Regardless of how this national health-care drama unfolds, people with epilepsy need to understand their current health-care options and make the most of them. The different types of health insurance are discussed in more detail in Chapter 18.

WHAT KIND OF DOCTOR IS BEST?

In the past, you could go to almost any doctor for most health problems. Now there are physicians who specialize in every imaginable medical problem, including epilepsy.

No one kind of doctor is best for all problems. People with epilepsy need two types of health care: (1) overall care to prevent and treat general medical problems, and (2) specialized care for epilepsy.

There is great value in having one doctor who supervises health care for you and your family. He or she can direct you through the health-care system, referring you to specialists when necessary. Physicians who help patients stay healthy and care for all types of medical problems are called generalists or family practice doctors.

General physicians who are a bit more specialized include pediatricians, who see patients under the age of 21; internists, who diagnose and treat problems in adults but don't perform surgery; and gerontologists, who primarily see patients over age 65. These doctors can diagnose and treat a great number of common illnesses. When a patient requires diagnosis or treatment for a more serious or a less-common problem, they should discuss the problem with or refer the patient to a physician who specializes in that disease or disorder.

Neurologists are physicians who specialize in treating diseases of the brain or other parts of the nervous system. They treat epilepsy, Alzheimer's disease, Parkinson's disease, and multiple sclerosis, as well as many other diseases and disorders. To qualify as a neurologist, a doctor must have several years of special training after medical school and must pass an examination given by the American Board of Psychiatry and Neurology.

Some neurologists concentrate on helping only patients with epilepsy. These "epileptologists" belong to professional epilepsy associations, such as the American Epilepsy Society, and usually also work closely with the public Epilepsy Foundation of America (EFA) and its local affiliate.

Making the Choice

How you choose a doctor or doctors to provide each type of care will depend on where you live, how you will pay for the care, and, possibly, how difficult your epilepsy is to control. Let's look at how each of these variables can affect your choice of doctors.

For regular medical care, you will, of course, want to establish a relationship with a doctor who is convenient to your home. If you live in a rural area you may have few choices, but your doctor should still be able to consult with a neurologist. Also, it may be well worth your time to travel to a university medical center or other large clinic for regular evaluations of how well your epilepsy is being controlled.

If you live in a city you will have many doctors to choose among. If you have indemnity (traditional) health insurance, or if you are going to pay for the care yourself, you can choose freely among the doctors in your area. You may look for a general physician in a medical center or at a university, where neurologists or epileptologists may also be accessible. The best way to find a good doctor is to ask your friends and neighbors for recommendations, and if you feel uncomfortable or unhappy with a physician, you are free to search for another.

Many people can no longer choose doctors quite that freely, however. More and more Americans are relying on HMOs and PPOs to pay for both routine and specialty health care. And with that reliance comes less freedom of choice in selecting physicians, clinics, and hospitals. Usually, though, you will have enough freedom within your insurance plan to find good medical care, especially if you are willing to be assertive and to spend time in making a selection.

People with epilepsy should have some type of health insurance coverage. Many people with chronic diseases find that the quality of health insurance an employer provides is a major consideration when looking for a job. Be sure to find out if prior conditions such as epilepsy are covered by a prospective employer's plan.

If you are not already covered by your employer's health insurance plan or an individual policy, find out what types of coverage are available in your state (see Chapter 18). Check each plan carefully, asking very specific questions about what is covered and how much is paid for each service, such as prescriptions, laboratory charges, routine doctor visits, visits to a neurologist, psychological counseling, hospitalization, surgery, and inpatient diagnostic services.

Another very important question to ask is, "If I think I need to see a neurologist to improve the control of my epilepsy, will I be able to, and will the visit be paid for?" Many people with epilepsy receive excellent routine health care and epilepsy monitoring from general practice physicians. But it is important that they be able to see a neurologist if needed. It is also important that the generalist be able to consult with a neurologist in making a diagnosis, prescribing treatment, and evaluating epilepsy control. This has become a problem in some health insurance plans, especially HMOs that restrict members to seeing certain doctors. In an effort to keep costs low, some HMOs will only pay for specialty care or service if one of their general practice doctors approves.

If you are not satisfied with your access to a neurologist, or if you are not sure that your doctor is communicating with a neurologist, you should ask your doctor about his knowledge in this area. Find out how much training in epilepsy care your doctor has had. Ask about recent epilepsy updates he or she has attended or read. These questions are not a challenge or threat, but rather a sign that you want to make sure you are getting the best possible epilepsy treatment.

If your insurance plan limits your access to specialized care, express your dissatisfaction to plan representatives. Start with your doctor, but realize that he or she may have little control over the type of coverage you have. Pursue your questions and concerns with your employer, and with representatives of your health insurance plan, such as the clinic business office, the customer relations department, and as far up the chain of authority as you have to go to gain satisfaction. If you are convinced that you have a reasonable request for quality health care, don't take no for an answer.

Finding Epilepsy Care

The EFA is a good source of information about neurologists and epileptologists in your area. If possible, attend local EFA meetings and volunteer your help. It is a great way to stay aware of advances in epilepsy treatment and to contribute to good epilepsy care and research. You will also be able to meet other people with epilepsy, who may be of help in solving problems or finding a good doctor. (See Chapter 19 for more information about the EFA.)

Most neurologists will be able to provide excellent care in all areas of epilepsy diagnosis and treatment. However, neurologists provide care in several different settings, which may affect the quality of care you receive. Some neurologists work alone, seeing patients in a private office. Others work in a larger office with other neurologists and possibly nurse-clinicians, who can provide education and spend additional time discussing health problems. Some neurologists work in large medical centers, which could meet almost every conceivable medical need you might have.

Each of these settings has good and bad points, and you need to find the one that works for you. Factors to consider in making a choice are:

- Length of time needed to get an appointment
- Telephone access to nurse-clinician or neurologist for help, especially in an emergency
- Willingness of neurologist to work with your regular doctor to monitor epilepsy control
- Feeling that your individual needs and preferences are considered and that you are part of the team working together to control your epilepsy
- Satisfaction that your epilepsy needs were met and questions answered at each visit
- Availability of laboratory services for evaluation of your treatment
- Ability to provide for other needs related to epilepsy, such as education, psychological and social counseling, financial assistance or advice, and help in working within the requirements of your health insurance plan
- Knowledge and effectiveness of the doctor treating you.

In some cities, special epilepsy centers have been established. These centers bring together epileptologists, nurse-clinicians, nurse-educators, psychologists, pharmacists, laboratory technicians, and other professionals, who work with patients and family members as a team to provide the comprehensive services often needed for optimal epilepsy care. Some have national reputations, which you could find out about from the EFA or the National Institutes of Health in Bethesda, Maryland.

An epilepsy center is likely to be the most experienced in managing difficult cases of epilepsy. These centers are often affiliated with a large university or medical center, where extensive diagnostic procedures can be done, and where more complex drug combinations can be monitored and surgical treatment considered. They are also usually involved in research, including clinical trials of new drugs that may improve epilepsy control. You should ask if the epilepsy center is a member of the National Association of Epilepsy Centers and meets the association's guidelines.

Don't Settle for Less Than You Deserve

Never stop evaluating your satisfaction with your general health care and the control of your epilepsy. There is always something that can be done differently, either by you or by your doctor. The next chapter provides some hints for making the most of your relationships with the people who provide your health care.

5

How to Be an Effective Member of Your Health-Care Team

Connie G. Frazer, R.N., and Robert J. Gumnit, M.D.

Many people take a passive approach when dealing with physicians and nurses. They act the way they think "good" patients should, sitting quietly while being examined, responding briefly to any questions they are asked, and leaving with a prescription for medicine or "orders" from the doctor. They behave as if their health belongs to the doctor, not to them. As a result, the doctor and nurse have only the patient's body to work with, not a whole person who can describe problems and help plan solutions. The most important member of the health-care team is missing an actively participating patient.

Reading this book shows that you want to be an active member of the team dealing with your epilepsy. Learning about the disorder will help you to become an informed patient—a vital step in controlling any chronic disorder. This chapter will help you use your knowledge and your problem-solving skills to become an active participant of your health-care team.

ARE YOU A MEMBER OF YOUR HEALTH-CARE TEAM?

You have to make a sincere effort to become an effective member of this team, since its success depends to a great extent on information provided by you and actions taken by you. Doing your best to report seizures accurately, along with any side-effects from medications, and general health problems, makes it possible for the rest of the team to develop a plan that best meets your needs and concerns. By following that plan, and by openly discussing any problems it presents or changes you think would improve it, you will be doing your part to achieve the best possible seizure control.

How do you feel about your health-care team? Answering some pertinent questions about your care will help you to evaluate it.

Ask yourself the following questions about your health-care professionals:

- Do you feel comfortable talking with your doctor and nurses?
- Do you have confidence in their professional skills in treating epilepsy, and in their ability to refer you to others for specialized care?
- Have they provided you with understandable educational information about epilepsy?
- Do they involve you in decision-making and planning, or do they just give instructions without asking how you feel about the way things are going?
- Do they take time to answer your questions, and do they talk to you using terms you can understand?
- Can you reach your nurse or doctor to ask questions and report problems?
- Are you satisfied with your epilepsy control?

Next, ask these questions about yourself.

- Do you understand all the services your health-care team can provide, and do you know whom to contact for what?
- Are you on time for appointments?
- Do you prepare for the visits by keeping good records and writing down the questions you want to ask?
- Are you honest and complete when presenting information and discussing problems?
- Do you take the time to learn about epilepsy as educational materials are presented?
- Do you take someone with you, if you need help describing seizures or understanding instructions?
- Do you listen carefully to instructions and write down information you might forget?
- Do you take your medications on time and follow other parts of your health plan?
- Do you ask for help when you need it for medical, emotional, social, or financial reasons?
- Are you satisfied with your epilepsy control?

The last question in both lists is the key one in evaluating your team. If you are truly satisfied that everything possible has been done to maximize your epilepsy control, then there is no need to change. (Of course, you may feel other areas of your health could be improved. If so, use the questions to evaluate those concerns.)

If you are like most people, however, there are several areas in which your health-care team could be improved. Here are some suggestions for improving your relationship with each team member.

IS YOUR RELATIONSHIP WITH YOUR DOCTOR SATISFACTORY?

Probably the most common complaints patients have are that physicians don't spend enough time with them and don't listen carefully enough to their questions or concerns. If you feel this way, don't assume that you have an uncaring doctor. There may be several reasons for a visit that feels rushed, and there are several things you can do to make better use of your doctor's time.

First, keep in mind that if you are feeling fine and there are no problems with your epilepsy control, you don't need to take much of your doctor's time. A quick exam and "Keep up the good work" are all you need.

But if you do have some questions to ask or problems to discuss, plan your visit carefully. When you make an appointment, explain why you are coming. Schedule visits well in advance if possible. A busy clinic may not be able to schedule you for a routine visit for two weeks or a month. But in a crisis, you should always be able to see a doctor or nurse-clinician or be referred elsewhere to have the problem taken care of.

A first visit requires 45 minutes to an hour. Not all this time will be with the doctor; you may also see a nurse-clinician, have blood drawn, and see some educational materials. Make the most of this first visit by making sure to have all your medical records transferred, or better yet, pick them up and bring them with you. Arrive early to allow time to fill out new patient forms and medical history questionnaires. Be sure to tell the nurse and doctor if you have a hearing or sight problem, don't read well, don't understand English well, or if you have any other problem that might interfere with your participation on the health-care team. There is always something that can be done to help increase your participation.

If you have financial questions about your care, ask to see the business manager or other appropriate person. Most clinics will help you to file insurance claims, and will help by scheduling reasonable payment plans. If a private clinic has accepted you as a patient and you later become unable to afford care there, that clinic has an ethical obligation to make sure that you receive care at a public facility.

Bring a written list of any questions, and ask them first of the nurse, generally the person most appropriate to provide such information. The best way to get a good start with your health-care team is to show them that you are prepared to use their time wisely.

If you are coming back for a routine clinic visit, expect to spend about 15–20 minutes. Again, make a list of questions, and ask the nurse or nurse-clinician which ones he or she can answer and which ones to ask the doctor. Then, when the doctor comes in to see you, mention that you have a few questions to ask at his convenience.

You should not hesitate to talk with your doctor, but neither should you feel free to chat *at length* about things not directly related to your health. When volunteering information, try to be as brief and clear as possible. If a family member or friend can explain things better, ask him to accompany you. Your doctor will appreciate any information that can help improve your epilepsy control and general health. Be a good listener, and expect your doctor to listen well in return. If your doctor is using terms you don't understand, ask for an explanation. Repeat in your own words what you are hearing; this will tell the doctor that you have heard and understood important information.

WHAT IF THINGS DON'T WORK OUT?

Probably the most difficult thing for a patient to ask a doctor for is for a referral to another physician. Whether for a second opinion, for specialty care, or to change doctors, it is common for the patient to feel awkward, as if this request is a criticism of his ability. There is no need to feel this way if you are convinced that your health care would be improved by seeing another doctor. Medical ethics require doctors to refer patients for a second opinion if asked.

Like any human relationship, sometimes a patient and a physician simply cannot communicate well or feel comfortable with each other. Whatever the reason for wanting to see another doctor, explain your desire to the doctor or nurse. Try to be matter-of-fact in stating your request, without being judgmental or hostile. Perhaps by explaining to the nurse what type of personality you would feel more comfortable with, you can be seen by another doctor at the same clinic. If presented honestly and politely, your request will almost certainly lead to a referral to a respected health-care team.

ARE YOU MAKING THE MOST OF YOUR NURSE?

Nurses are often the glue that holds the health-care team together. They can skillfully perform a variety of health-screening tests and procedures. They gather much of the information the doctor needs to make decisions. Nurses must also be skilled at communicating medical information to patients and making sure that the physician's instructions are understood.

In general, the nurse's job is to help you make the most of the time you spend with your doctor. To do that, she needs your help and cooperation. Tell the nurse the reason for your visit and express any special concerns you want to be sure the doctor is aware of. If, after you see the doctor, you have a question or remember something else you wanted to ask, tell the nurse. Your question will be addressed as soon as possible, but if it is a major but nonemergency problem you may have to make another appointment.

WHAT CAN THE NURSE-CLINICIAN DO FOR YOU?

As we explained in the last chapter, some clinics employ nurse-clinicians: registered nurses with special training in a specific area of medicine. The nurse-clinician can provide much of the routine care and exams usually done by doctors, freeing them to deal with more complicated problems.

The nurse-clinician can spend more time with you and can answer many of your questions. Your doctor will work closely with the nurse-clinician to determine what needs to be done at your visit and what changes, if any, need to be made in your epilepsy control plan. If the nurse-clinician has to pry information out of you, time will be wasted for both of you. By providing all the information your nurse-clinician asks for, you will be assured of a successful visit.

The nurse-clinician is also a good resource when calling in to the clinic with problems or questions about epilepsy. Rarely is it necessary to speak to a physician. The nurse-clinician will either provide a solution, consult with the doctor, or have him return your call if necessary.

WHO ELSE IS ON YOUR HEALTH-CARE TEAM?

There may be several other members of your health-care team to help you improve seizure control. Your pharmacist, for example, can do more than fill prescriptions. Questions about epilepsy medications, side-effects, interactions with over-the-counter medications, dosages, and generic versions of brand-name drugs may all be addressed by your pharmacist. (But never make any changes in your medications without first consulting your doctor.)

Social workers and psychologists can be extremely helpful, because epilepsy tends to affect all aspects of life. By getting help before financial or emotional problems become severe, you can greatly decrease your stress and the harmful impact on your life and those you love. These professionals will be discussed in later chapters.

The most enjoyable part of being a health-care professional is helping patients who want to do everything possible to get the most out of life. By conveying that type of spirit and attitude, you will become a real member of the team and greatly improve the quality of your care.

WESTERN IOWA TECH - LIBRARY

6

The Importance of Complete and Accurate Diagnosis

John R. Gates, M.D., and Robert J. Gumnit, M.D.

It is common to think of "the diagnosis" as the time a doctor said that you or a loved one has epilepsy. Actually, there is much more to a complete and accurate diagnosis. As described in Chapter 2, there is more than one type of epilepsy and more than one kind of seizure. In order to decide on the appropriate treatment to control seizures, the kind or kinds of seizures a person is having must first be determined.

Sometimes the diagnosis of epilepsy is very clear because there is a good description of the individual's seizure. If proper treatment is prescribed and no more seizures occur, there may be no need for extensive diagnostic tests. But if the diagnosis is not clear, and if the initial treatment does not prevent further seizures from occurring, further diagnostic tests will be necessary. These may even determine that the patient does not have epilepsy. This chapter will discuss the initial diagnosis of epilepsy, as well as various tests that can be done if the diagnosis is not clear.

WHY ARE THEY ASKING ALL THESE QUESTIONS?

When a person first has a seizure, it is likely to be a very distressing time for the family. If the seizure is severe, causing convulsions or unconsciousness, the person will probably be taken to a hospital emergency room. A first seizure usually lasts a little more than a minute, and the person and family might not be able to describe it very well. However, any description of behavior or feelings before, during, and after the seizure is very helpful.

If the seizure was severe, the patient will probably be admitted to the hospital for one to three days for observation and diagnostic tests. If it was not severe enough to bring the patient to the hospital, a diagnosis may be attempted in a doctor's office, or he may decide to hospitalize the patient for further care and diagnostic tests. Antiepileptic drug therapy may begin at once to avoid the potential danger of further seizures.

The first part of the diagnostic process is finding out the patient's and the family's complete medical history. Because epilepsy sometimes runs in families, it is important to provide as much information about the family as possible. The doctor or nurse may ask questions about the patient's behavior, problems with bedwetting, history of head injury, health problems as an infant, family health problems, mental health, and use of alcohol, street drugs, or medications.

The questions may not always seem to be related to epilepsy, but the answers can help a doctor familiar with the disorder to make a clear diagnosis. Withholding any information out of fear or embarrassment will often eliminate any chance of preventing more seizures.

The most useful information for the doctor is a clear and accurate description of the seizure. This is also the most difficult information to obtain.

After the medical history is gathered, the doctor will perform a complete physical examination, which will focus especially on the nervous system. He will do several tests that evaluate the condition of the nerves leading from the brain to different parts of the body.

WHAT IS AN EEG?

The most commonly used test to diagnose epilepsy is an EEG, or electroencephalographic examination, which can detect the very small amount of electricity given off by the brain. All living things generate small amounts of electricity, and the human brain creates electrical charges as activity takes place within it.

The EEG machine translates this brain electricity into a set of wavy lines. A neurologist can tell from the pattern of these lines if there is something wrong with a part of the patient's brain. Often, though, the EEG recording will look normal except during the time the patient is actually having a seizure. Initially, most EEG recording sessions are about 30 minutes long, but additional EEG recordings may be done for several hours. If the seizures occur many days apart, however, it may be hard to diagnose them using an EEG.

Having an EEG is a safe procedure and does not cause shock or discomfort. Also, it does not "read your thoughts," it merely records the electrical activity of your brain. The test may be given in a hospital or in a neurologist's office, in a room where the patient can relax during the test. Wires called *electrodes* are glued to the patient's scalp. There is a slight pinprick when each electrode is attached. The technologist doing the test may ask the patient to breathe rapidly at times and may shine a blinking light into the patient's eyes. A recording may also be made while the patient is sleeping.

WHAT IS THE PURPOSE OF A CT OR MRI SCAN?

Computed tomography, or CT scanning, is a special type of radiologic procedure that is used to take pictures of the brain. The CT scanner is a large machine that has a round opening for the patient's head. An X-ray camera just inside the opening revolves around the head, taking pictures of the brain at different angles and different depths. These X-ray pictures are then analyzed by the computer to show structures within the brain.

A CT scan is a painless procedure that takes about 15 minutes. A fluid called a *contrast medium* may be injected into the patient's arm. This fluid travels to the brain and makes the scan easier to read. All that is required of the patient is to relax and hold as still as possible while the scan is being taken.

By reading the CT scan, a doctor may be able to spot some damage inside the brain that could be generating abnormal electrical signals and causing seizures. Or, the CT scan may reveal a blood clot or tumor within the brain. If a tumor is detected, it is important to remember that most tumors are not cancerous. Many are abnormal clusters of tissue that can be surgically removed without any danger of spreading. Cancerous tumors can also often be effectively treated with surgery and radiation.

An even newer technology than the CT scan is magnetic resonance imaging (MRI), in which a huge magnet is used to create a magnetic field within the patient's body. This magnetic field is used to generate a picture of the inside of the body. When focused on the brain, the MRI computer generates pictures similar to a CT scan, but in more detail. The MRI may be used to obtain a better image of an abnormality detected on the CT scan. The CT scan and MRI look at the *structures* of the brain, while the EEG records its *function.*

An experimental technique called positron emission tomography, or PET scanning, is being used for research on the brain. It measures changes in the metabolism of brain cells. Although some promising results have been obtained, it is too soon to know how useful PET eventually will be.

WHAT CAN BLOOD AND URINE TESTS TELL ABOUT A SEIZURE?

Whether the patient is seen in the hospital or in a doctor's office, laboratory tests will be ordered to detect any problems that may have contributed to the seizure. These may include infection, organ failure, mineral imbalance, high or low blood sugar, or any other of a large number of abnormalities that show up in the blood or urine.

WHEN SHOULD MORE DIAGNOSTIC TESTS BE PURSUED?

If a diagnosis of epilepsy has been made and drug therapy started, but the seizures are not under control after three months, further diagnostic tests should be done. If a neurologist was not involved in the initial diagnosis, this is definitely a time to find one, preferably one who specializes in epilepsy.

The neurologist may repeat many of the diagnostic tests done earlier. This will be especially true in children, who are often more difficult to diagnose. The neurologist will be trying to clarify the seizure type to see if the appropriate medication is being used. Several different epilepsy medications may be tried, as will be discussed in the next chapter.

If antiepileptic medications do not control the seizures within nine months, the patient should be seen by a neurologist who specializes in treating epilepsy, at an epilepsy center. Specialized diagnostic tests will then be done to reevaluate the diagnosis. These will determine whether the person is experiencing psychogenic seizures (described in Chapter 2) or is one of a minority of people who have epileptic seizures that are especially difficult to control.

One group of tests that may be performed is known as a *neuropsychological examination.* These examine how different parts of the brain are performing and can help to localize any disease or disorder that may be present. Some of these tests study motor function (body movements), reaction time, planning abilities, memory and brain function.

The epileptologist may decide to hospitalize the person to perform intensive neurodiagnostic monitoring. Some hospitals have facilities and trained personnel to film the person with a video camera while an EEG is recorded for many hours. The patient stays in a comfortable room hooked up to an EEG, while a videocamera tapes all activity. Simultaneous video/EEG is the most accurate way to diagnose the type of seizure. Antiepileptic medications will be withdrawn before or during this time to make it more likely that a seizure will occur. When one or more seizures are recorded by this video/EEG recording, the epileptologist will be much more likely to make an accurate diagnosis. This is because the person's behavior can be matched to his brain function, showing what type of seizure is occurring.

Sometimes a technique called *telemetry* is used to try to record a seizure on EEG while the patient is given more freedom of movement in the hospital. In one type of telemetry, the patient has scalp electrodes placed on the head, which are connected to a device that amplifies the signals and sends them through a long cable to the EEG. This type of telemetry is used when the patient is at risk of falls or injury during seizures.

A second type of telemetry gives the patient more freedom. The electrodes are attached to an FM transmitter that sends the signals by radio waves to a receiver hooked up to the EEG. Telemetry can enable the patient to be monitored for as long as 72 hours at a time.

Some patients experience seizures only when they are going about their normal daily routine. In these cases, a less-effective but still useful system called ambulatory monitoring may be tried. The person wears a small, portable EEG recording device hooked to scalp electrodes. When a seizure occurs, the person pushes a button to mark where on the EEG it took place. This can provide a good EEG picture of a seizure, but the scalp electrodes often lose contact, and good recordings are not always obtained.

WHY IS DIAGNOSIS SOMETIMES SO COMPLICATED?

Epilepsy is a complex disorder that is often a mixture of more than one type of seizure. To treat all the patient's seizures properly, the doctor must find out which parts of the person's brain are affected and which type of seizure or seizures the person is having. Only then is it possible to develop a treatment strategy that will control the seizures to the greatest extent possible. The next two chapters will describe the two most common treatments for epilepsy: medications and surgery.

7

Medications: The First Choice in Epilepsy Therapy

Ilo E. Leppik, M.D., and Robert J. Gumnit, M.D.

The prescription of antiepileptic medications is by far the most commonly used method to treat epilepsy. The initial treatment plan must be closely monitored at first to make sure that it meets an individual's needs. While the specific medications prescribed may differ somewhat from person to person, the goal is always to select the medication that will completely control seizures, while having no effect on general well-being.

It is not always possible to achieve this goal with the first attempt, but cooperation between the patient and the treatment team usually makes it possible to arrive at a good result. This chapter describes how you can help design your medication therapy and participate in adjusting it to meet your needs.

HOW DOES A PHYSICIAN DECIDE WHICH MEDICATION TO PRESCRIBE?

More than 20 different medications are currently available to treat a patient with epilepsy, and new ones are continually being evaluated in clinical trials to see if they might be useful. In practice, however, three medications are used to treat the majority of people with epilepsy, and several others are used frequently.

The most common antiepileptic medications are listed in Table 7-1. As you can see, certain substances are used to prevent certain types of seizures. This is why a complete and accurate diagnosis is so important, as was discussed in Chapter 6. Your doctor will select from the medications that are effective in controlling your type (or types) of seizure. Other factors that will be considered include: (1) medication allergies you've had in the past, (2) your age, (3) your ability to conceive (some may cause birth defects), and (4) your ability to pay (some medications cost a lot more than others).

Overall, the medications available to treat epilepsy are effective, but their effectiveness varies from one individual to another. Therefore, it is

Table 7-1. *Most Commonly Used Anticonvulsant Drugs
Approved in the United States and
Specified Seizure Type*

Drug	U.S. trade name	Seizure type	Primary or secondary drug
Carbamazepine	Tegretol®	Generalized tonic–clonic	Primary
		Simple partial	Primary
		Complex partial	Primary
Clonazepam	Klonopin®	Simple partial	Secondary
		Complex partial	Secondary
		Myoclonic	Primary
		Absence	Secondary
Ethosuximide	Zarontin®	Absence	Primary
Mephobarbital	Mebaral®	Simple partial	Primary
		Complex partial	Secondary
		Generalized tonic–clonic	Secondary
Phenobarbital	Luminal®	Generalized tonic–clonic	Secondary
		Simple partial	Primary
		Complex partial	Secondary
Phenytoin	Dilantin®	Generalized tonic–clonic	Primary
		Simple partial	Primary
		Complex partial	Primary
Primidone	Mysoline®	Generalized tonic–clonic	Secondary
		Simple partial	Secondary
		Complex partial	Secondary
Valproic acid	Depakene®	Absence	Primary
		Generalized tonic–clonic	Primary
		Myoclonic	Primary
		Complex partial	Secondary
Divalproex sodium (slow release form of valproic acid)	Depakote®	Absence	Primary
		Generalized tonic–clonic	Primary
		Myoclonic	Primary
		Complex partial	Secondary

necessary to try the medication most likely to control your seizures. Your doctor will prescribe the recommended daily dosage, which is the amount of the substance that is known to be safe and effective for someone your age and weight.

He will also tell you when to take the medication. The total daily dosage of some antiepileptic medications can be taken once a day, while with others the daily dosage must be divided into two to four doses. This is because the medications have different *"half-lives,"* the time it takes for half of the dose to be eliminated from the body. Medications with longer half-lives can be taken once or twice a day, because they are removed from the body more slowly and effective levels remain in the body for a longer time. Those with shorter half-lives must be taken more often, because they are effective for shorter periods.

The different half-lives of antiepileptic medications allow your doctor some flexibility in prescribing a medication that will be convenient for you to take. However, sometimes seizure control is not achieved with the most convenient dosage schedule. In that case, you may have to take a higher dosage, which may have to be split into several pills taken at different times of the day. Also, some people have seizures at about the same time of day. In these cases, the doctor will want the person to take the medication at a time that will make the drug most effective.

It is very important to take the pills at the time or times prescribed by your doctor. You should therefore set up a system to help you remember to take them. Many people find a weekly pill holder very useful. This box contains several compartments for each day of the week. By filling it on Sunday, for example, you will be able to tell whether or not you have taken the pill or pills for each day. Or try keeping a calendar with your medication timetable on the refrigerator or other prominent place, and check off each time you take a pill.

Do your best to take your medication on time. But if you forget, take the missed dose as soon as you realize it, or take it together with the next scheduled dose if necessary. Ask your doctor or nurse for help in setting up a system, and discuss what you should do in case you forget to take a dose.

You should also discuss with your doctor the possibility of side-effects from your medication. Like all other medications, each antiepileptic drug has side-effects that might occur in some people but not in others. If there is too much of a substance in a person's system, he or she may feel unusually tired, unsteady, confused, or nauseated. These and other mild side-effects of the common antiepileptic medications are listed in Tables 7-2 and 7-3. They have occurred in a minority of the thousands of people taking the medications, and, of course, no one person would have all these symptoms. And most people will not have any side-effects. But if you do experience any of these side-effects or any other unusual feelings or symptoms, tell your doctor. It is usually possible to eliminate them by changing the medication or the schedule on which it is taken.

It is also possible, but much less common, for an individual to experience an allergic reaction to an antiepileptic medication, usually a skin rash. Or extra sensitivity to a certain substance may cause severe drowsiness or mental confusion. If these types of side-effects occur, inform your

Table 7-2. *Side-Effects That May Be Seen with Commonly Used Antiepileptic Medications*

Frequent (10–30% of persons may have these); dose-related (can be reduced by reducing the amount of medicine)
Dizziness
Tiredness
Sleepiness
Loss of balance
Change in memory
Nausea

Unusual (less than 1 or 2%), but may be fatal, and medicine must be stopped
Skin rash (allergic reaction)
Liver failure
Anemia
Bleeding problems
Very low white blood cell count

Table 7-3. *Side-Effects Specific to Each of the Medicines*

Carbamazepine
  Low sodium levels with blood count (serious)
Phenytoin
  Acne
  Hair growth
  Gum growth
Valproate
  Hair loss
  Weight gain
  Irregular menstrual periods

doctor. A different medication can be prescribed to avoid these unacceptable reactions.

After your doctor has prescribed a medication for you to take one or more times each day, you or your family will need to keep track of how effective it is. Until the seizures are well under control, it is very important to keep a detailed diary of any seizures that occur and any side-effects experienced by the person with epilepsy. Don't try to memorize this information! Write it down! Be as detailed as possible in describing the seizures and side-effects, including time of day and what the person was doing when the seizure or side-effect occurred.

WHAT IF THE MEDICATION DOES NOT CONTROL MY SEIZURES?

It is not uncommon for the first medication to control a person's seizures only partially. This is where the diary kept by the patient or family plays a major role in working toward seizure control. It is especially important to be completely honest in reporting whether pills were taken at the scheduled times, or whether a dose was forgotten. Your doctor will be grateful for this information—not angry. Ask for suggestions if you can't find a system for remembering to take your pills.

Depending on the antiepileptic medication chosen, it will take from several days to a few weeks for the substance to reach a maximum level of effectiveness. Then, depending on how often you have seizures, you and your doctor can begin to evaluate the effect of the therapy. If your seizures are not controlled by the starting dosage of the medication, your doctor will increase the dosage gradually. Frequent laboratory blood tests may be performed to make sure that the desired amount of the substance is in your body. Since each individual's body handles each drug differently, testing your blood levels allows your doctor to make sure that the desired amount of medication is remaining in your body.

As your doctor increases the dosage, it may reach a point of *toxicity,* when side-effects occur because too much of the substance is in your system. If the medication has not had any effect on your seizures, your doctor will start you on another medication. You will probably be asked to decrease gradually the amount of the first medication you were taking, to give the second medication time to build up to effective blood levels. Then, you and your doctor will follow the same process in evaluating the effectiveness of the second medication.

If the first medication reduced your seizures somewhat before toxicity occurred, your doctor may decide to *add* a second medication. You will continue to take the first medication, but at a dosage one level below that at which you experienced side-effects. The second drug will be added to your medication schedule, possibly at different times of day than the first drug. If adding this second medication does not achieve seizure control, your doctor will gradually increase its dosage until either control or toxicity is reached.

Frequent testing of the amount of medication in your blood (blood levels) is especially important when taking two antiepileptic medications, because the substances can interact with each other in different ways in different people. The only way to know how much of each medication is in the blood at any time is to perform a laboratory blood test. Drug interactions can be complicated, and your physician may decide to consult with or refer you to a neurologist or epileptologist.

Most people with epilepsy can achieve seizure control with just one medication, if it is properly prescribed and taken. But some people may experience more than one type of seizure or have seizures that are difficult to control. These people may be helped by taking two medications, and in rare cases more than two medications may be prescribed. The four keys to finding the right medication or the right combination of medications are:

- Taking the right medication at the right time
- Having blood levels tested frequently
- Keeping good records of seizures and side-effects
- Working closely with an experienced epilepsy team

HOW WILL MY EPILEPSY MEDICATIONS AFFECT OTHER MEDICATIONS AND ALCOHOL?

Check with your doctor before taking any other type of medication, including those you can buy without a prescription. Most over-the-counter medications such as aspirin, acetaminophen (Tylenol), and cold medicines can be taken occasionally without affecting seizure control, but check with your doctor or pharmacist.

Whenever you see a doctor or dentist for any reason, be sure to tell the nurse and doctor that you are taking antiepileptic medication. This will help the doctor if it is necessary to prescribe another type of medication. For example, some antibiotics, especially erythromycin, might have to be avoided because they can double or triple the effect of some antiepileptic medications.

Moderate consumption of alcohol—an occasional social drink—usually will not cause problems for a person with epilepsy. However, heavy alcohol consumption is one of the most frequent reasons people with epilepsy are seen in hospital emergency rooms. Also, street drugs such as cocaine, barbiturates (downers), and amphetamines (speed) can cause severe and dangerous seizures. A person with epilepsy who abuses alcohol or other drugs must receive help for that problem before antiepileptic medications can be effective.

ARE THERE OTHER WAYS ANTIEPILEPTIC MEDICATIONS CAN AFFECT MY HEALTH?

If antiepileptic medications are properly prescribed and monitored to prevent side-effects, there usually will be very few other effects on your health. An unusual effect that has gotten quite a bit of attention—more than it deserves, actually—is a slight overgrowth of the gums in one-fourth of the people who take Dilantin, one of the most widely prescribed antiepileptic medications. This can be controlled by proper daily brushing and flossing, and by regular visits to a dentist.

As mentioned earlier, antiepileptic medications may cause birth defects, so it is important for a woman to tell her doctor if there is a chance she may become pregnant. The unborn baby can be affected by medications even before a woman knows she is pregnant, so it is important to plan ahead. If sexually active, a woman should discuss birth control or appropriate changes in her medications with her doctor. See Chapter 16 for special concerns involving marriage, sex, and having children.

CAN I SAVE MONEY BY SUBSTITUTING A GENERIC BRAND FOR MY MEDICATION?

Never make a change in your antiepileptic medication—either in brand name or dosage—without first checking with the doctor who prescribed it. Antiepileptic medications are especially sensitive to steps taken in the manufacturing process. For example, the way they are made into pills can have a significant effect on how they are released in your body. In 1987, the Food and Drug Administration (FDA) issued a warning that one of the generic types of antiepileptic medications was failing to control seizures in people who had been well controlled when taking the brand name of that same substance.

If your seizures are hard to control, it is important that you not switch from brand name to generic, or from one generic manufacturer to another, without special supervision. The differences allowed by law in the manufacturing of medications may be too much for you. It is important to realize that the distributor of generic medications may put the same label on medications from different manufacturers, and that even the pharmacist dispensing the medicine may be unaware of this. Record the lot number and distributor's name each time you get a generic medication, in case questions arise or you have unexpected seizures.

Your doctor can help you to make changes safely to reduce the cost of your therapy. It may be possible to save money by taking a generic form of your medication, but your physician must be involved in this decision. You can often save money on brand names or generics by searching for the pharmacy with the best price. If your doctor prescribes a generic form, you should be able to purchase it at nearly half the cost of the brand name of the same medication. You have to shop around, though, because some pharmacies make a large profit on generic drugs by not passing along as much of their own discount. By working with your epilepsy team to find out which form of a substance will work for you, and then by finding the least expensive pharmacy, you can get the lowest price possible on your medication.

To avoid confusion and the possibility of receiving the wrong medication, keep a card in your purse or wallet with all the information on your epilepsy medication. *Don't allow anyone but your doctor to make any kinds of substitutions in your prescription.* If the pharmacist has any questions about your prescription, he should call your doctor or nurse.

IS IT REALLY IMPORTANT TO FOLLOW MY MEDICATION SCHEDULE EVERY DAY?

An international conference of epilepsy experts was recently held to discuss the problem of patient compliance. These experts estimated that anywhere from 30% to 50% of people with epilepsy do not take their antiepileptic medications as scheduled. This was thought to be a major reason for lack of control of seizures and disability due to epilepsy.

Everyone will forget to take a pill once in a while, but there is no excuse for an occasional lapse becoming a general lack of effort that affects seizure control. No number of visits to a doctor and no type of diagnostic test can be effective if medications are not taken as scheduled. It is not the doctor or nurse who is being let down if the therapy is not followed, it is the person with epilepsy. Remember, *you* are the most important part of the epilepsy control team.

WHAT IF MEDICATIONS DON'T CONTROL MY SEIZURES?

If your doctor is continuing to make medication adjustments, is testing your blood levels frequently, and is consulting with an epilepsy specialist on your case, do your best to be patient and follow the therapy closely. It may take three months to test each medication fully—longer if you experience seizures only rarely.

However, if medications do not control your seizures, you should consider being evaluated at a comprehensive epilepsy program. The health professionals at these programs have the knowledge, experience, and medical equipment needed to evaluate cases of epilepsy that are difficult to control. They may want to hospitalize you to perform the extensive diagnostic tests discussed in Chapter 6. They can also offer the newest types of antiepileptic medications, with close monitoring and evaluation of blood levels. It is not always possible to eliminate seizures completely, but health professionals will help you get the best possible seizure control and improve your ability to cope in all areas of your life.

Surgery is another possible option that may result from an extensive hospital evaluation. This is a relatively new therapy for epilepsy, which has helped to reduce or eliminate seizures in a growing number of people who are not helped by medications. The next chapter will explain what types of surgery have been effective in controlling seizures, and how individuals with epilepsy are evaluated to find out if surgery might help them.

8

Surgical Options

John R. Gates, M.D., Robert E. Maxwell, M.D., and Robert J. Gumnit, M.D.

Thanks to advances in technology and increasing knowledge about the brain, surgery is becoming a more common and safer option for treating epilepsy. Surgery is the first choice for treating epilepsy when seizures are caused by a brain tumor or by a head injury that can be surgically repaired. Surgery also may become an option if seizures cannot be controlled after repeated attempts at medication therapy, or if the medications cause unacceptable side-effects. Surgical treatment of epilepsy should not be taken lightly, but it should also not be dismissed without weighing its benefits against its risks. The possible benefits and risks must be assessed for each individual.

Determining if a patient can benefit from surgery is a demanding and difficult task. The skills of several disciplines must be brought together in a coordinated fashion. Neurologists or neurosurgeons who specialize in epilepsy (epileptologists) usually head the team. In addition to a neurologist and a neurosurgeon, a neuropsychologist and a neuroradiologist are usually included. Most patients will utilize the services of a social worker or counseling psychologist, and occasionally a psychiatrist as well. Many tests will be performed.

Patients and their families will have many questions and concerns during the time surgery is being considered. It is very important to have all questions answered and concerns addressed. This will help everyone participate in making a decision if the team determines that surgery should be considered. Once it is decided to have surgery, or not to, everyone involved can best help the person with epilepsy by showing a positive attitude about the future.

This chapter describes the most common types of surgery done to help people with epilepsy. It is only an introduction to this subject, however. Family members and individuals with epilepsy considering surgery should seek out additional sources and ask their doctors for more information about their specific situations.

IS EPILEPSY SURGERY A NEW TECHNIQUE?

No. The first American report of surgical attempts to treat epilepsy was in 1828, when Dr. Benjamin Dudley, a university professor in Kentucky, reported successfully removing skull fragments and blood clots from the brains of people who suffered head accidents that resulted in epileptic seizures. At that time, there was no anesthesia and operating rooms were quite primitive and unsterile. But remarkably, all five of Dudley's patients survived and did well. In contrast, half of the patients died in similar operations in the United States and Europe for the rest of the 19th century.

The next type of surgery for epilepsy involved the removal of a brain tumor. This was first done successfully in 1884 by a German surgeon, Dr. Rickman J. Godlee. It was quite remarkable because there was then no way of taking a picture of the brain to locate the tumor. The patient's tumor was diagnosed by Dr. Hughes Bennett, a neurologist, using knowledge gained by German researchers studying the brains of animals. They found that by electrically stimulating parts of the brain, convulsions could be caused in precise parts of the body. They mapped out which parts of the brain controlled which parts of the body. This made it possible for Bennett to find out where the patient's tumor was by observing the signs and symptoms that it caused.

The modern era of epilepsy surgery began with the introduction of electroencephalography, or EEG. In Chapter 6 we described how the EEG is used to diagnose epilepsy. The EEG was developed during the 1930s and 1940s, and it first began to be used to locate the focus of epileptic seizures in the 1950s. Dr. Wilder Penfield, a Canadian neurosurgeon, is often said to be the father of modern epilepsy surgery. He established and directed the Montreal Neurological Institute, where Dr. Herbert Jasper showed that EEG recordings could be used to locate the focus, or area of the brain in which a patient's seizures begin. Penfield was one of the first surgeons to operate primarily to control seizures, removing a part of the brain to reduce successfully the severity of the patient's seizures without damaging vital functions.

Today, epilepsy surgery is performed by specialized teams throughout the world. Advances in the fields of neurology and neurosurgery, in diagnostic equipment, in operating room technology, and in postsurgical care have all contributed to make surgery a reasonably safe and effective option for some people with epilepsy.

WHEN IS SURGERY AN APPROPRIATE TREATMENT FOR EPILEPSY?

Surgery is appropriate when, after extensive diagnostic testing and consultation about a patient's epilepsy, the team determines that it is the method most likely to improve the person's life. Of course, even if the doctors believe it is appropriate, the final decision is up to the patient, or to the family if the patient is a child or is incapable of participating in the decision-making.

There are many possible reasons neurosurgeons may decide that surgery is appropriate. Perhaps the patient has a bone fragment, blood clot, or tumor that is affecting part of the brain. In a case such as this, surgery may be much less risky than leaving the problem as it is. Modern operating techniques often make it possible to repair a brain injury or remove a tumor without seriously affecting the patient's brain function.

Surgery may also be appropriate if neurologists have tried all possible options for medication therapy and the person's seizures are intractable—out of control for six months or more. Sometimes medications will control a person's seizures, but only at dosages that make it impossible for him to function normally. This would be another reason to consider surgery.

However, not everyone with intractable seizures is a candidate for surgery. It is hard to make general estimates about the percentage of these people who may be helped by surgery. This is because the likelihood that surgery will help depends on what type of seizures the person has. It is estimated that about 25% of people with epilepsy have seizures that are difficult to control with medications, and that almost half of them (10% of people with epilepsy) are thought to have seizures that may be reduced in severity or eliminated with surgery.

The types of seizures most likely to be helped by surgery are those that begin in a small area, or *focus,* in the brain. If the team can locate this focus with EEG and other diagnostic tests, and if they determine that this brain tissue does not serve a vital function, such as speech or memory, they may recommend surgery to remove the area.

Another type of surgery is sometimes performed when a person's seizures start in one area but spread rapidly throughout the brain. If not controlled, these seizures can cause dangerous falls. It is sometimes possible to stop the seizures from spreading by cutting part of the tissue that connects the two halves of the brain. This surgery and the type above are explained further in the next section.

WHAT ARE THE COMMON TYPES OF EPILEPSY SURGERY?

Temporal Lobectomy

The most common type of epilepsy surgery involves stopping complex partial seizures (see definition of seizures in Chapter 2) by removing a part of the brain called the temporal lobe. This is called temporal lobectomy ("ectomy" refers to surgical removal).

The brain has two halves, or hemispheres. Each half has a temporal lobe on the side of the brain. One of the temporal lobes, usually the left, is dominant for speech, meaning that it has more control of language functions than the other lobe. The temporal lobe also controls memory and the ability to express thoughts in words.

About 70% of people who have a temporal lobectomy in a leading epilepsy center are seizure-free after surgery. Many surgical patients will still have to take medications to control their seizures. There is about a 3–5% risk of a partial loss of vision, motor function, memory, or speech after a temporal lobectomy.

Corpus Callosotomy

The second most common type of surgery for epilepsy involves partly disconnecting the two cerebral hemispheres, or halves, of the brain. The two hemispheres are interconnected by a bundle of nerve fibers called the corpus callosum. This bundle of fibers acts as a kind of bridge that allows electrical activity to spread from one hemisphere of the brain to the other. Some people have seizures that start in one hemisphere and then spread through the corpus callosum to the other. These generalized seizures can be very dangerous, causing the person to fall without warning.

The operation to cut part of the corpus callosum is called a corpus callosotomy. Epileptologists have found that if they cut about two-thirds of the corpus callosum, they can often prevent or reduce the number of seizures that spread to the second hemisphere. This results in the patient having predominantly partial seizures, which are less dangerous, because they usually don't cause falls. Few patients who undergo a corpus callosotomy will be seizure-free after surgery. Most will have much less severe seizures that can be controlled with medications. Sometimes a second operation to complete the division of the corpus callosum is necessary if the first is not successful. There is about a 10% risk of some complication occurring as a result of a corpus callosotomy.

Other types of surgery for epilepsy are less common. One example is removal of the entire nondominant hemisphere. This is usually done in young children with significant paralysis of one arm and hand, and who have many severe generalized seizures every day. These problems make life very dangerous and prevent children's development. Remarkably, it has been found that these children can be successfully rehabilitated, because the dominant hemisphere can be trained to take much of the control of both sides of the body. The child usually experiences only a slight worsening of the paralysis on the side of the body that was controlled by the hemisphere removed in surgery.

WHAT TESTS WILL BE DONE BEFORE SURGERY IS RECOMMENDED?

Before a team at an epilepsy center decides that surgery is an appropriate treatment for a particular patient, they will usually repeat all of the diagnostic tests described in Chapter 6. They will first want to make sure that the patient really does have intractable seizures, i.e., seizures that cannot be controlled in other ways. Then they will want to know as much about the seizures as possible. This can only be done by video/EEG recording of several seizures. If a focus in the mesial portion of the temporal lobe is suspected, this is followed by even more extensive EEG recording, which may include placing sphenoidal electrodes into the depths of the tissue at the base of the skull, over the sphenoid bone. This is necessary because the skull blocks or weakens some of the faint, abnormal electrical signals from deep within the brain. CT and MRI may also be done to prodvide information about brain structures (see Chapter 6).

Also, it may be possible to determine what part of a person's brain is affected by having him do a number of neuropsychological tests. These include muscle movements and mental tests that require the involvement of certain parts of the brain. How he completes the tests may indicate that a specific part of the brain is not functioning correctly, even when he is not having a seizure.

Several additional diagnostic tests will be performed before surgery. A *cerebral angiogram* will be done to show the surgeon where blood vessels are located in the patient's brain. A special fluid is inserted into an artery; when this fluid reaches the blood vessels in the patient's brain, a picture is taken with film that shows the fluid within the brain blood vessels.

Usually at the time the angiogram is performed, a test called a Wada test (or intracarotid amytal) will be done. This involves injecting a fluid called sodium amobarbital into the main arteries on either side of the neck, the carotid arteries. This shows the neurologist which side of the brain is dominant for speech and memory, because when the fluid is injected into the artery that delivers blood to the dominant hemisphere the patient will be temporarily unable to speak, or may have memory problems. The injection also may reveal on which hemisphere of the brain the seizure focus is, because when the artery on that side is injected, seizure activity may be temporarily blocked.

Doctors may also inject doses of a depressant medication called sodium pentothal into one of the patient's veins. This affects EEG activity in very characteristic ways that help identify whether a person's generalized seizures start in one or more areas of the brain and then spread.

Based on these tests, the doctors and the patient (or family) will decide whether to go ahead with surgery. If surgery is to be performed, rehabilitation specialists will do additional diagnostic tests. They will want to measure the person's abilities in areas such as speech, motor function, vocational aptitude, and other types of functional areas. This information can then be used to compare his or her abilities in the months and years following surgery.

If the team is confident on the basis of video/EEG recordings and other tests that the surgery can be safely performed, then all that remains is to schedule the operation. All sections of the corpus callosum and most temporal lobectomies can be performed without resorting to an additional operation to insert electrodes into (depth electrodes) or on top of (subdural electrodes) the brain.

Occasionally the information from scalp recordings is not clear enough to decide where to operate. There may be a question about which temporal lobe to remove (right or left) or whether the seizures arise in the frontal or temporal lobe. In that case, depth electrodes will be placed in the frontal and temporal lobes on each side in an operation using a special device called a stereotactic frame. This enables the surgeon to place the electrodes in the precise part of the brain to be studied. The operation usually can be performed under a local anesthetic, that is, without putting the patient to sleep. Extensive video/EEG recordings will be taken to record several seizures, enough so that the doctors are confident they know where to operate. This may take anywhere from one to three weeks. Following this, the electrodes are removed (a relatively simple and painless procedure) and the patient discharged. If surgery is to be performed, the surgeon will let the brain heal for a month or more before readmitting the patient for removal of brain tissue.

If the focus appears to be located near vital portions of the cortex of the brain (for example, speech, movement, feeling areas) extensive caution is needed. This usually occurs if the focus is quite far back in the temporal or frontal lobes. In that case, an initial operation is performed under general anesthesia (patient completely unconscious) to insert a subdural grid containing many electrodes, which actually stay inside the head resting against the brain for about two weeks. A subdural grid looks like a plastic card covered with metal dots. During the initial operation, the neurosurgeon carefully places the subdural grid under the outer covering of the patient's brain, directly over the part that seems to be the origin of the seizures. Then the surgeon closes the patient's scalp, leaving the grid temporarily inside the skull, with the leads protruding through the scalp so they can be hooked up to an EEG machine.

After surgery, the patient may feel nauseous for a few hours, although sometimes that will last for the first few days. There is some headache, which slowly improves. Most patients are reasonably comfortable with the grid or depth electrodes in place and do not require a pain killer.

In the days following surgery, the patient will be monitored closely by EEG. The grid must be kept in place until enough seizures take place to indicate with certainty which area of the brain is involved. Anticonvulsant medications may be withdrawn to allow seizures to take place, but the patient is given pain medication and kept as comfortable as possible during this time.

Additional testing will be done by stimulating parts of the patient's brain while EEG monitoring is taking place, during which the patient will be asked to move the arms and legs and perform simple mental tests. This testing helps the neurosurgeon to detect which sections of the brain are involved in important functions such as speech, memory, and sight.

Testing done with the subdural grid in place may show that a patient is a good candidate for removal of affected brain tissue. If so, the neurosurgeon will discuss the surgery with the patient and family and will plan for a second operation. During this operation, the subdural grid will be removed and brain tissue will be removed to attempt to eliminate the area causing the seizures and thereby improve the patient's seizure control.

However, the testing may also show that the affected brain tissue is in an area that controls an important function. It may be too risky to try to remove part of this brain tissue. In this case, a second operation will still be performed to remove the subdural grid, but no brain tissue will be removed, and the person would not be expected to have any change in seizure frequency.

HOW CAN THE PATIENT PREPARE FOR SURGERY?

The best way to prepare for surgery is to find out as much as possible about the surgery and its possible outcomes. The nurses, doctors, psychologists, and social workers who are part of the team can help answer questions about the diagnostic tests, about the surgery itself, and about the recovery period. This may be a very stressful time for the patient and family, and it can be very helpful to talk about that stress with a professional counselor who is familiar with patients undergoing brain surgery.

The best way to find out about possible outcomes of the surgery is to ask the neurosurgeon or nurse if it would be possible to talk with others who have had the same type of surgery. Ask to talk with a person who has had a great outcome, a person who has had a satisfactory outcome, and one who has had a poor outcome. By hearing about the different possible outcomes of the surgery and about how each individual feels about the surgery, the patient and family can make a decision based on the best information available. This will also prepare them for the recovery process and rehabilitation following surgery.

Some patients and families make the mistake of expecting too much from surgery. It is natural to feel that if a major problem in life, such as epilepsy, were to be suddenly removed, everything would be perfect. This is not true for epilepsy or for other life problems. There will always be other challenges that must be faced, and a person cannot change overnight.

Even if surgery does result in a seizure-free life, seizure-free is not worry-free. Some patients become depressed because they expect surgery magically to change their lives. Talking with other people who have had surgery for epilepsy will provide some of this realism. And meeting with a psychologist can help a person analyze the situation and prepare to make the best out of whatever happens.

When a decision is made to go ahead with surgery, everyone involved must do his best to think positively. It is natural to be afraid and to worry. Focusing on a positive result will help everyone get through the waiting period and will help motivate the patient for the postsurgical recovery.

WHAT WILL HAPPEN DURING AND AFTER SURGERY?

The patient will usually be admitted to the hospital the day before surgery. Routine blood and urine tests and a chest X-ray will be done to make sure he is healthy enough to undergo surgery. The patient's head will be shaved to provide a sterile area for the operation. He will not be able to drink or eat anything after midnight if the surgery is to be done under general anesthesia.

The type of anesthesia that is used depends on the type of surgery and, in some cases, on the preference of the surgical team. Some surgeons prefer to have the patient completely asleep during the surgery to allow more intricate and lengthy procedures.

The surgery will take several hours, and then the patient will be moved to a recovery area. Here he will be closely monitored until the anesthesia wears off. Then it will be possible for a few family members to visit. It is not uncommon to have quite a bit of facial bruising and swelling following surgery. The patient will be very tired for the next few days and may not want to do anything. The length of time spent in the hospital depends on the type of surgery and how quickly the patient recovers. Many of the diagnostic tests done before surgery may be repeated in the days following to evaluate its effects. Rehabilitation will begin in the hospital and a schedule of visits will be set up for the next few months.

When released from the hospital, the patient will continue the process of recovery and rehabilitation. Recovery after temporal lobectomy usually takes a few weeks, while it occasionally takes as long as six months to fully recover from corpus callosotomy. Working with a neurological rehabilitation unit can be extremely helpful, but much of the rehabilitation will be carried out at home with the help of family and friends. Recovery from temporal lobectomy is usually uneventful, although some patients experience headaches. However, a few patients who required a complete section of the corpus callosum undergo personality changes and throw temper tantrums in the weeks following surgery. Basic behaviors such as eating, drinking, and bladder control may have to be relearned. Speech may be difficult and mental processes slowed. Most patients who only have an anterior two-thirds section have a much easier recovery period. It is very important that the patient and family realize that these problems are usually temporary. By following the recovery schedule set up by the neurological team, basic skills can be relearned and behavior will return to normal. It is natural to try to push too hard and expect too much during the recovery period. Remind each other that this is a gradual process and that the best result will come from working together and being patient with each other. It can sometimes take a couple of years to heal completely.

The ideal outcome of epilepsy surgery is to eliminate seizures and use of medications. This is not a very realistic goal for most patients, however. A more realistic outcome is for the seizures to be less severe and be more easily controlled with medications. Some patients have a few seizures one or two months after surgery and then medications bring them under control.

If seizures are still not controlled, it may be possible to repeat the surgery after about six months, but this is rarely done. New medications are being discovered and tested in clinical trials, and one of these may be helpful. By staying aware of progress in epilepsy therapies, the patient and family can keep working toward a better future.

Epilepsy surgery will not magically solve a person's problems, but in most cases it will give the person a better chance for a more normal life. Surgery provides new opportunities, and it is up to the person and family to take it from there.

9

Being Prepared: First Aid for Seizures

John R. Gates, M.D., and Tess Sierzant, R.N.

Seeing a seizure for the first time can be quite shocking, especially when you don't understand what is happening and don't know what to do. The Epilepsy Foundation of America is working hard to teach the public how to help someone who is having a seizure, but there is still much ignorance. People with epilepsy and their families and friends can help bridge this gap in understanding.

It is very important that a few simple first-aid steps are known by everyone who spends time with a person who has epilepsy. This includes family members, other relatives, friends, teachers, babysitters, coworkers, teammates, etc. Wearing a medical-alert bracelet or necklace is a good way for a person with epilepsy to increase the chance of a helpful response to a seizure from the public.

The first part of this chapter provides some basic first-aid steps to take when someone is having a seizure. The latter part explains how to recognize an emergency situation called *status epilepticus.*

HOW CAN YOU TELL WHEN A PERSON IS HAVING A SEIZURE?

Three general types of seizures that can be distinguished by the person's behavior when the seizure occurs are as follows.

Generalized Tonic–Clonic Seizures

This is the type most familiar to the public, because it is the most dramatic. The person may fall, stiffen, make jerking movements, and may bite his tongue. The skin may turn pale or bluish because of difficulty breathing, and loss of bladder or bowel control may occur. The person will be unresponsive during the seizure and afterwards may be confused, disoriented, and sleepy.

Complex Partial Seizures

This is the most common type of seizure. Unfortunately, it is sometimes mistaken for drunken or drugged behavior. The person may appear to be awake but will speak nonsense and will not respond to questioning. Many types of behavior may be seen, but most commonly the person may have a glassy stare, fail to respond correctly or at all to questions, move about aimlessly, make lip-smacking or chewing motions, fidget with clothes, and may become angry and aggressive if restrained.

Absence Seizure

This type occurs mostly in children. It often goes unnoticed because the only outward sign may be rapid blinking or a blank stare. The person appears to be awake but is briefly unaware of surroundings and events. He may miss parts of information, such as school lessons, or may have gaps in memory of recent events.

WHAT CAN BE DONE FOR A PERSON HAVING A SEIZURE?

For all seizure types, the best thing to do is remain calm. If other people are present, reassure them about the seizure. Unless one of them has more experience with seizures, tell them that you will help the person. Different kinds of seizures require different kinds of help, but in general the objective is simply to remove any dangerous objects from the vicinity and wait until the seizure is over.

Keep in mind that a seizure cannot be stopped once it starts. What you *can* do is to help keep the person from being injured, and reassure him afterwards. Don't try to shake a person out of a complex partial seizure, and don't try to restrain someone having a tonic–clonic seizure.

The most common myth about generalized tonic–clonic seizures, in which the person has convulsions and sometimes turns blue from interrupted breathing, is that he is in danger of swallowing his tongue. *This is not true.* It is actually impossible to swallow the tongue. Don't put anything in the person's mouth! All this does is cause broken teeth and injured jaws, as well as finger injuries to the well-intentioned giver of first aid. It also reduces the person's ability to breathe. Wait until the seizure is over and the body begins to relax, then turn him on his side to maintain a clear airway and allow saliva to dribble out.

Remain with the person during and after the seizure, preventing injury and providing reassurance by speaking softly. If the seizure stops and the person regains awareness, it is usually not necessary to call an ambulance. Check to see if he is wearing a medical-alert bracelet or necklace with instructions about whom to call. Tell the person what happened. Ask if there is anything you can do, such as helping him get home or providing a description of the seizure.

The following are specific steps to take for each type of seizure.

Generalized Tonic–Clonic Seizure

1. Help the person into a lying position and put something soft under the head.
2. Remove eyeglasses and loosen any tight clothing if possible.
3. Clear the area of hard or sharp objects, such as furniture.
4. Do not force anything into the mouth.
5. Do not try to restrain the person—let the seizure run its course.
6. After the seizure, turn him on one side to let saliva drain from the mouth and allow the tongue to fall forward and open the airway.
7. The person may awaken confused. Be calm and reassure the person that everything is all right.
8. Do not give him anything to eat or drink until fully awake.
9. Stay with him until fully alert, then ask if there is anything you can do to help.

Complex Partial Seizures

1. If the person wanders, do not try to stop or restrain him.
2. Try to remove harmful objects from the person's path, and gently coax him away from stairs or other hazards. Physically intervene only if it is absolutely necessary to prevent an accident. Get help if you are alone and the person is aggressive.
3. Talk calmly. Do not agitate the person by shaking or shouting. He may become angry or aggressive if interfered with.
4. After the seizure, the person may be confused. Stay with him until fully alert. Ask if there is any way you can help.

Absence Seizures

1. These seizures are usually very brief, so just try to be aware of when a seizure may have occurred.
2. Provide any missing information and help the person get back into the lesson, conversation, or activity.

WHEN DOES A SEIZURE BECOME A MEDICAL EMERGENCY?

Although most seizures end in less than a minute or two and require no medical attention, on rare occasions it is necessary to call for an ambulance. For example, if someone is injured during a seizure or does not start breathing within two minutes after it, call an ambulance and begin treating the injury or providing mouth-to-mouth resuscitation. If an injury is not apparent, ask the person if you should call an ambulance or a doctor when he is fully alert.

Another reason to call an ambulance is if a tonic–clonic seizure does not stop after three or more minutes, or if another seizure starts very soon after the first one ends. *Status epilepticus,* or continuous seizure state, is a life-threatening medical emergency if continuous tonic–clonic seizures occur. The person needs special medication as quickly as possible to stop the seizure and prevent harm.

WHAT CAUSES STATUS EPILEPTICUS?

The most common cause of status epilepticus is when a person stops taking antiepileptic medication for some reason or does not take it often enough to maintain effective blood levels. Another less common cause is an illness with fever or infection. These conditions sometimes cause the body to remove the medication from the blood too quickly to be effective.

Status epilepticus is treated in the hospital by doing whatever is necessary to help the patient breathe and stopping the seizures with intravenously administered medications. Blood tests are performed to find the cause of this episode, such as low level of antiepileptic medication or low glucose. If the cause is found to be a low blood level of antiepileptic medication, the patient will be given an intravenous injection of the medication. Other causes will be treated appropriately, and the patient will be watched carefully until the seizures have stopped. The doctor who supervises his epilepsy therapy should be contacted.

IS IT POSSIBLE TO LESSEN THE EMBARRASSMENT AND PUBLIC FUSS THAT A SEIZURE CAN CAUSE?

Yes, through public education about epilepsy. When people understand something, they are less likely to fear or ridicule it. Prepare friends and relatives for what to do when a seizure occurs. Calmly explain seizures and dispel myths when they occur in public, so that we can all decrease the possible harm and embarrassment to the person with epilepsy.

10

Seizures in Newborns and Infants

Richard V. Andrews, M.D.

Epileptic seizures are not unusual during the first month of life (the newborn, or "neonatal," period) and the first year of life (infancy). The occurrence of a seizure during this time presents special problems for both parents and health-care providers. The events are often quite frightening, and at times are quite frustrating as well. Anxiety and frustration can be minimized if everyone involved understands the nature, causes, and effects of seizures in newborns and infants. This chapter will provide a general explanation that will help parents participate in the evaluation and treatment of their child.

Seizures in newborns and infants are often difficult to recognize, since they may not appear to be markedly different from normal behavior. As a result, they often go undiagnosed unless they occur frequently or dramatically. Parents sometimes feel guilty if they have not recognized the events as being seizures from the very start. However, seizures can be very subtle, or quite brief, and even nurses and doctors may have difficulty recognizing their true nature. Often the diagnosis is made only when looking back, after considerable time has passed.

Prompt evaluation is very important for a newborn or infant who may have had a seizure. It may be a symptom of a serious problem that should be corrected quickly. Or it may indicate a more complex problem that requires further diagnostic testing and therapy. Seizures are occasionally the first sign of an extremely serious disease process.

Because it is often difficult to diagnose seizures in newborns and infants, both extensive overtreatment and undertreatment are common. EEG monitoring has been used in research centers to help investigate seizures. This fairly expensive technology is now beginning to be used for clinical care in some newborn intensive care units. However, it is difficult to interpret newborn EEG tracings. Many EEG patterns that would be considered markedly abnormal in older children are absolutely normal for a newborn's stage of brain development. Unless the doctor has an extensive familiarity with newborn EEG, misinterpretation can result in misdiagnosis and inappropriate management. Much new knowledge needs to be gained with the use of EEG monitoring and other techniques in order to make a significant impact on the diagnosis of epileptic seizures in newborns.

The best clue that a baby's movements are epileptic is the stereotyped, repetitive nature of most seizure movements. Although the events may be brief, they often look very similar, like "variations on a theme." We have very little idea how common newborn or infant seizures really are, because so many go undiagnosed, are misdiagnosed, or are isolated events and never recur. However, it is not safe to assume that a single seizure is nothing to worry about and that the problem will go away by itself.

Family members should understand that a baby suspected of having a seizure needs an immediate evaluation, since an underlying cause may be very quickly correctable. That does not necessarily mean that emergency *treatment* is indicated. Starting treatment with antiepileptic medications without a clear diagnosis is a mistake, because many nonepileptic movements and events will stop also as a result of this treatment. If the nature of a movement is not clear, observation may be the first step, together with a general evaluation to be sure the baby is in no immediate danger.

Evaluation of a suspected seizure starts with a detailed history: exactly what happened, what the baby did, what went on immediately before the event and for several hours and days beforehand. A full account of the pregnancy, labor, delivery, and development to date is also important. A clear, accurate description of the suspected seizure event is of prime importance, because the entire diagnostic and therapeutic approach hinges on it.

An infant having an epileptic seizure presents a diagnostic challenge, because the brain's development is incomplete and it still lacks many functions. Thus, many brain functions cannot be evaluated during a neurologic examination of an infant. Some testing procedures may therefore need to be done that might not be necessary in an older child.

A seizure is a cause for concern, but no early, preconceived notions should be assumed about what this will mean for the baby's health. One should not "assume the worst," but should await the outcome of the evaluation. Many different processes can result in a loss of normal control of brain function. Finding a correctable or treatable cause is what the diagnostic workup is really all about. Some parts of the search are very easy, other parts are quite difficult, laborious, and expensive. Nonetheless, it all starts with an accurate description in everyday common terms of exactly what happened.

WHAT CAN CAUSE A BABY TO HAVE A SEIZURE?

The nature of a baby's brain and brain function makes it somewhat easier for a seizure to be triggered by a slight change in the brain's environment. The most common causes of seizures in both newborns and infants are an imbalance in body chemistry, an infection, or a suddenly developing fever. Some of the causes are very serious, but many babies have seizures that eventually disappear on their own with no adverse effects.

One particularly serious type of problem results from brain injury occurring just before or during the birth process. If severe, this "perinatal brain injury" can cause very severe and uncontrollable seizures. These seizures are actually related to an imbalance of body chemistry. During the stress of the birth process, the baby's brain may have been exposed to an abnormal supply of glucose (blood sugar) or oxygen. Slight lack or excess of these important nutrients, or of minerals such as sodium and potassium, can upset the brain chemistry enough to trigger a seizure.

An infection can also put extra stress on a baby and trigger a seizure. Even minor infections often cause a baby to develop a striking fever, with body temperature rising quite rapidly. It is thought that this rapid rise in body temperature is what actually triggers a "febrile seizure." A seizure may also be the first sign of a more serious infection of the central nervous system, such as meningitis or encephalitis, which requires immediate treatment.

Other, rare problems can also cause a baby to have a seizure. These include several types of disorders of metabolism and digestion that may be "congenital," which means the baby was born with the problem. Some babies are born without the ability to make enough of one of the many chemicals that brain cells need to be able to function correctly. These are called "inborn errors of metabolism." They may be related to the way the body metabolizes fatty acids, how the body makes and processes proteins, or to the way the body digests and processes sugars. These processes are complicated, and their diagnosis and treatment can be extensive and costly.

WHAT DO SEIZURES LOOK LIKE IN NEWBORNS?

Identifying seizures in newborns can be difficult, since they are usually somewhat subtle. Babies rarely have tonic–clonic convulsions, in which the person first stiffens and then has rhythmic jerky movements involving the whole body. A young baby's brain is not developed enough to cause this kind of seizure.

The only outward sign of a seizure in a baby may be uninterruptible staring, unusual rhythmic eye movements, sudden loss of body tone, or rhythmic movements of one or two limbs that cannot be stopped by repositioning the baby or holding the limb. In one common type, the baby's legs are flexed up against the body very rapidly. In general, a seizure may be occurring if a baby is doing something that the baby cannot be distracted from by holding, touching, or repositioning, or if the baby has sudden jerky movements. Any of these signs would be good reasons to have the baby examined. It is important to keep in mind, however, that many movements may appear to be seizures, but after an examination and medical tests they may turn out to be something else.

Breath-holding spells (called apneic spells) are very rarely epileptic. These events need to be investigated, but usually another cause is found. It is not unusual for true breath-holding spells to start well before the baby is one year of age.

In recent years, there have been dramatic advances in our ability to keep premature and sick newborns alive, especially in hospitals with a neonatal intensive care unit (NICU). There are many reasons babies spend time in an NICU, ranging from precautionary monitoring of vital signs to advanced life support after a severe brain injury at birth.

Seizures may result from many types of birth injuries. These include bleeding within the brain (intraventricular hemorrhage), blockage of blood flow in the vessels leading to the brain (stroke), or not getting enough oxygen to the brain (hypoxia). They may also result from problems that can occur during fetal development of organs such as the heart, kidneys, and lungs. These problems that are present at birth are called congenital disorders. A congenital problem may be the underlying cause of a birth injury, such as when a heart defect results in not enough oxygen being delivered to the brain.

The most useful method for diagnosing newborn seizures is to monitor the electrical activity in the baby's brain. This is done with ongoing EEG monitoring, which means the EEG is recorded continuously rather than for a half hour or hour at a time. Many NICUs now have the capability to do this type of monitoring. It is very important to have the EEG analyzed by a neurologist who is familiar with seizures and with the EEGs of newborns and infants. Specific patterns of electrical activity are associated with different stages of development of a baby's brain. Seizure activity on a newborn's EEG is often somewhat different from that of an older infant, just as a child's EEG is different from that of an adult.

The fact that a baby has a neonatal seizure does not necessarily mean the baby will have brain damage or other neurological problems. These seizures can be provoked by medically correctable problems, treatment for which may end the baby's seizures and lead to a good outcome. Doctors may give the baby antiepileptic medication in order to prevent repeated seizures that may harm the baby's health. If the cause of the seizures can be found and corrected, the medication is usually withdrawn after a brief time.

New mothers are now being sent home from the hospital with their babies much earlier than in the recent past. This is not necessarily bad, if the mother or someone else is able to care for the baby and any other children. It does mean, however, that some things that used to be detected in the hospital may be missed due to the shorter observation period. It is especially important, therefore, for new parents to question anything that appears to be abnormal in their baby during the first few days and weeks after birth. Everything that has already been described about seizures in sick newborns also applies to healthy newborns, especially to a premature infant or one who has had any kind of difficulty at birth.

Another cause for seizures, mentioned briefly above, is the rapid development of a fever. Most febrile seizures are benign, meaning that they do little or no harm. They are not usually associated with ongoing problems, including the development of epilepsy. A baby who has one or more febrile seizures is usually not at any greater risk for developing other health problems.

Seizures may occur as a result of a viral illness that causes vomiting or diarrhea. The baby may develop an imbalance of minerals, or of total body water, all of which are important in maintaining normal nerve function. In addition, the body fluids must maintain the correct level of acid–base balance, or pH level. An imbalance or lack of a number of other nutrients or enzymes can also trigger seizures. Babies, in general, develop these imbalances faster than older children and adults. Usually, a detailed history can help the doctor determine if one of these imbalances is the cause of a seizure, and appropriate treatment can take place.

Although most seizures in newborns and infants do little or no harm, it is not uncommon for epilepsy to appear before the age of one year. Even if the disorder does not really become apparent until the child is older, a family will often remember a seizure that occurred early in the child's life. It is important to make a note of events such as this, as they can help with the diagnosis of problems that may occur later in life.

WHAT DOES A SEIZURE LOOK LIKE IN AN INFANT?

In older babies closer to one year of age, seizures are often more dramatic. They still usually last less than about five minutes or so. Usually the baby will have some staring from which it cannot be distracted. There may be some repetitive movements of limbs, and they can be quite violent. Breathing may be uncoordinated and cause the baby to turn pale or slightly blue.

It is important not to panic or do anything harmful if this occurs. Such acts as trying to restrain movements or force the baby's mouth open can do much harm and are unlikely to do any good. First aid for an infant's seizure is much the same as for an older child or adult (see Chapter 9). This means that all that is necessary is to place the infant in a safe position and wait for the seizure to end.

If the seizure does not end after about five to seven minutes, or if repeated seizures occur, emergency assistance may be necessary. If a seizure ends in a relatively brief time, parents may want to take the infant to an emergency room for an evaluation. This may not be necessary if the child is already being treated for seizures, but in any case the doctor should certainly be informed that a seizure occurred. Thus, while panic should definitely be avoided, it is appropriate to inform a doctor when a seizure occurs, and to pursue expert evaluation if it is not already under way.

HOW ARE SEIZURES DIAGNOSED IN NEWBORNS AND INFANTS?

Diagnosis of a baby's seizures often includes tests of urine and blood, and sometimes of spinal fluid. A neurologic exam is essential in order to check the baby's awareness, alertness, response to noise, and other signs of central nervous system function.

The doctor may then decide to do brain imaging such as CT or MRI scanning, or cranial ultrasound, in addition to an EEG (see Chapter 6 for a description of these tests). These tests are more frequently done in children under one year of age, and they may not be necessary in older children. This is because the nervous system is more developed in older children, which makes it possible to evaluate their brain function with a thorough neurologic exam.

WHAT TYPE OF DOCTOR SHOULD CARE FOR AN INFANT WITH A SEIZURE DISORDER?

A child under one year of age should be cared for by a pediatrician familiar with childhood neurologic problems and with seizures occurring during the newborn period. The pediatrician may be assisted by consultation with a pediatric neurologist. Such a specialist can be found in most major cities, especially those with major medical centers. The pediatric neurologist does not need to be the infant's primary doctor. It is usually helpful to have an expert evaluate the child initially, and then for the family to regularly visit a pediatrician who can continue to consult with the neurologist.

It may be expensive to have an infant evaluated by a pediatric neurologist, especially if the parents do not have health insurance to cover such services. Making this investment early, however, can often save a great deal of money, anxiety, and ongoing major medical problems that can affect the baby's future. A good long talk with a reassuring pediatric neurologist can often help parents be more comfortable in managing their child's problem. This can help prevent panic-stricken visits to the emergency room every time the child has an unusual event of any kind. It can also help involve the parents in finding the best possible treatment for the baby's seizures, and help the family know when to seek appropriate medical care and when they can handle a situation on their own.

HOW ARE INFANTS' SEIZURES TREATED?

Managing an infant with multiple seizures can be quite difficult, because at this age a child is developing rapidly both physically and mentally. It is very important that they be treated appropriately—not unnecessarily. Some medications can seriously affect development. It is important that if medication is used, the type and dose should be those least likely to interfere with a child's development and outcome. A pediatric neurologist can work closely with a pediatrician to maintain a safe and effective treatment regimen for the patient. This may include developmental assistance programs and other help when necessary.

If no seizures occur for several years, and the EEG has returned to normal, it may be possible to gradually withdraw the medication to see if the child is still susceptible to seizures. This should be done with the close supervision of a pediatric neurologist familiar with childhood epilepsy. It is certainly not appropriate for everyone who had seizures as a newborn or infant.

In spite of the frightening aspects of seizures in newborns and infants, these children can often develop normally and enjoy happy, productive, full lives. This is most likely if the child and family have the benefit of an appropriate health-care team. Treatment of childhood seizures and challenges for parents of a child with epilepsy are discussed in the next two chapters.

11

Treating Childhood Seizures

Frank J. Ritter, M.D., and Lisa M. Butler, R.N.

This chapter answers questions we are often asked by parents. Sometimes we can't answer with absolute certainty, because there are many things medical experts still don't understand about seizures. We can, however, provide information and suggestions that will help parents work with their child's health-care team.

IS IT COMMON FOR A CHILD TO HAVE SEIZURES?

Yes, it is quite common for children to have seizures. About one in 20 children has at least one febrile seizure, the kind of seizures caused by fever. About half of these children will go on to have more febrile seizures. Over a lifetime, one in 11 people will have a seizure. However, only three in 100 people experiences recurrent seizures that lead to a diagnosis of epilepsy.

WHAT IS THE DIFFERENCE BETWEEN A SEIZURE DISORDER AND EPILEPSY?

These terms are often mistakenly used to refer to anyone who has had a seizure. First of all, some people, especially children, will have only one seizure in their entire life, and it is incorrect to say that they have a seizure disorder or epilepsy. The terms seizure disorder and epilepsy both refer to someone who has had more than one seizure on more than one occasion, but the two disorders are quite different.

The difference is related to what is causing the seizures. If a short-term, treatable cause such as a fever, infection, or chemical imbalance can be identified as the reason for repeated seizures, then the problem would be described as a seizure disorder. A seizure disorder will usually go away with proper treatment or with time. Sometimes, however, seizures may continue even after proper treatment of the underlying cause. If this is the case, a diagnosis of epilepsy would be made.

Epilepsy would be the diagnosis if a child has two or more seizures that are not provoked by a temporary, treatable cause. In this case, an antiepileptic medication would probably be prescribed to try to prevent additional seizures.

WHAT CAUSES SEIZURES IN CHILDHOOD?

Childhood seizures can be caused by many things, including fevers, infections, chemical imbalances, head injury, low blood sugar, temporary lack of oxygen, or for reasons that can't be identified. Most of the seizures that occur in childhood are benign, which means they will do little or no harm, but sometimes a seizure can be a sign of a serious problem. This is why every seizure needs to be evaluated and treatment begun if a cause is found.

The most common cause of childhood seizures is a fever. The febrile convulsions that result are usually benign, and are not usually treated with antiepileptic medications. However, an immediate evaluation is necessary after a child's first seizure, even if the parents suspect that a fever is the cause. The fever may be related to an infection that must be treated promptly to prevent serious problems. If febrile seizures continue to occur, the parents should report them to the child's doctor. Unless directed otherwise, it is usually not necessary to take the child in to be examined after each seizure. If the fever persists, it can be treated with a nonaspirin product such as acetaminophen (Tylenol or similar product) and with a cool water bath. It is seldom possible to prevent a febrile seizure, so parents should not feel guilty if seizures do occur.

Febrile seizures often run in families, although it is possible that parents will be unaware of any relatives who had the problem as children. Some families seem to inherit a lower threshold for febrile seizures, but the seizures may not have been documented in the medical record or discussed with relatives. If parents are aware of a familial link, they should discuss it with the physician, because this can make the diagnosis more certain. Everyone outgrows febrile seizures, if fevers are indeed the true cause of the seizures. In a few cases, usually in children under the age of five, a seizure with a fever may be the first sign of the onset of epilepsy. It is rare for a child older than five to have a true febrile seizure for the first time.

Another common cause of childhood seizures is abnormal electrical activity in the brain that results in absence seizures. This is a type of epileptic seizure in which the child may become briefly unaware of his or her surroundings and may blink rapidly. The seizures (sometimes called "spells") may occur many times during the day. The child is usually motionless, unaware of surroundings, and fails to respond to voices or other outside stimuli. Like febrile seizures, absence seizures tend to run in families and they occur almost exclusively in childhood. They usually begin between the ages of 3 and 10 and almost always disappear before the child reaches adulthood.

Because absence seizures are triggered by abnormal brain functioning, they are classified as an epileptic seizure. If a child has absence seizures, a doctor will prescribe medication. Sometimes an absence seizure occurs before a seizure in which convulsions occur. About 50% of children with absence seizures will also have at least one generalized tonic seizure.

In most cases of childhood epilepsy, doctors are unable to identify a cause. There may have been an injury or oxygen shortage before or at birth, an undetected infection, a developmental abnormality, or some other past occurrence that resulted in the abnormal brain function. While it may not be possible to identify the original cause, it is important for every child who has had two or three seizures to be evaluated to diagnose what type of seizures they are having (see Chapters 2 and 6). A thorough diagnosis is crucial because a number of physical and psychological disorders can mimic epilepsy.

How extensive a child's diagnostic evaluation needs to be depends on how much information is available about the child's seizures, whether there is a clear family pattern of seizure activity, whether the seizures are controlled with medications without unacceptable side-effects, and whether the child has any associated problems such as developmental delay, mental retardation, movement disorder, or abnormality found in a careful neurological examination. Parents are doctors' greatest allies in this process, because the information they provide makes the biggest difference in what the doctor can do for their child.

CAN A CHILD DIE DURING A SEIZURE?

This is a common question asked by parents who are understandably afraid that the convulsions and temporary abnormal breathing could cause their child's death. In fact, in a survey of parents whose children had seizures, 80% of them thought at first that the child was dying. Fortunately, it is rare for a child to die because of a seizure. Many people fear the old myth of swallowing one's tongue during a seizure, but this is impossible (except in a child with a severe cleft palate).

If simple first-aid steps are taken (see Chapter 9), little harm ordinarily comes from a seizure. The most common threats to a child during a seizure are being injured by hard or sharp objects, and choking on saliva or vomit. An emergency situation may develop if the child goes into prolonged seizure activity called status epilepticus. If this is a recurrent problem for your child, your doctor can instruct you in the use of rectal anticonvulsant in emergencies.

WHAT ARE THE CHANCES THAT A CHILD WILL OUTGROW EPILEPSY?

Children do tend to outgrow certain types of epilepsy, but it is difficult to say for sure if and when a specific child might outgrow the disorder. Chances are greater if the epilepsy is a type that runs in families. Also, as we stated above, almost everyone outgrows febrile and absence seizures. The cause of the seizures also helps predict whether the child will outgrow them.

Even if it is unlikely that a child will outgrow his epilepsy, parents can be encouraged by the new, more effective medications and other treatments that are resulting from epilepsy research (see Chapter 21). As medical researchers gain more knowledge about the brain, there is greater hope that a cure for some or all types of epilepsy will be found.

WHAT TYPE OF DOCTOR SHOULD A CHILD WITH EPILEPSY SEE?

The choice of a doctor or doctors depends on whether or not the child's seizures are under control. All children need to see a pediatrician or family practice doctor for regular check-ups and for minor illnesses. This doctor may also be able to manage a child's epilepsy, depending on how difficult the seizures are to control.

We recommend that a child who has had two or more seizures, but whose epilepsy is now under control, should see a pediatric neurologist at least once. Most major medical centers have a pediatric neurologist on staff. This doctor will most likely be a specialist in childhood epilepsy. The pediatric neurologist can evaluate the child's medication plan and general well-being, and can answer any questions the parents may have about their child's epilepsy. Then, depending on the pediatric neurologist's recommendation, the child may be followed by the pediatrician or family physician. Repeat visits to the pediatric neurologist may be necessary if problems arise, and the child's doctor can consult the pediatric neurologist whenever necessary.

If a child's seizures are *not* under control, or if unacceptable medication side-effects occur, we recommend that families find a pediatric neurologist to manage the child's epilepsy. This doctor will be familiar with all the options for a child whose seizures are difficult to control. Not all children's seizures can be prevented or controlled, but they can almost always be reduced in severity. This may take six months to a year or more, as the neurologist tries different antiepileptic medications or different combinations of medications. It helps for parents to remain patient and carry out the doctor's instructions during this time. Parents need to take an active role in reporting seizures and medication problems to their doctor. If the family is not happy with what is being accomplished, they should ask to see a different neurologist, or to visit a center that specializes in managing epilepsy.

HOW IS CHILDHOOD EPILEPSY TREATED?

If a diagnosis of epilepsy is made, almost all children will be placed on a daily dose of one or more antiepileptic medications (see Chapter 7). Most will respond to the first medication tried, but some will not. If this is the case, a second medication can be added. If this is effective, the first medication should be gradually discontinued to see if the seizures can be controlled by the second medication alone. The objectives of this treatment evaluation are to control the child's seizures with the fewest number of medications, the lowest effective dose(s), and the least possible side-effects. If this goal is not reached after trying two or three medications, the child should probably see a pediatric neurologist or visit an epilepsy center.

All medications have side-effects. Doctors refer to side-effects as drug toxicity. The dose of drug and the blood level of drug that results in toxicity are highly individual. So it is important to carefully evaluate each child's blood levels of medications, and how well the child is functioning to determine what is an effective and nontoxic dose. The blood level of medication measured in the laboratory is extremely helpful in determining how to adjust dosages for your child. However, whether the child is seizure-free and does not have side-effects from the medications must be determined by observation. This is where the family is an extremely valuable part of the health-care team. Some types of medication toxicity are detected by blood tests, so it is extremely important that these tests are done as directed by the physician.

With antiepileptic medications, the most common dosage-related side-effects are drowsiness, behavioral change, sleep disorders, or change in appetite. Unsteady walking and vomiting may also occur. It is usually possible to find a medication or a dose that results in good seizure control with an acceptable level of side-effects. The child and parents must decide what type and severity of side-effects are unacceptable. Be fussy—don't settle for poor seizure control or side-effects that prevent the child from learning and participating in normal activities.

The most important thing for parents and children to realize about antiepileptic medications is that to be effective they must be taken in the doses and at the times prescribed. Make sure you follow the doctor's directions about whether the child is to take the medication before or after meals. Develop a system for keeping track of each day's doses, such as placing the pills in a pill container with a section for each day. If the child must take medication at school, meet with the school nurse to discuss his medication needs and other matters related to epilepsy (more about this in the next chapter). Most schools will not allow a child to take medication without some adult supervision, but it is important that the child be given as much responsibility as possible.

WHAT IF A CHILD MISSES A DOSE OR TAKES A DOUBLE DOSE?

Missing one dose of medication or taking a double dose (one parent gives the medication and the other parent or grandparent unknowingly repeats it, for example) will probably not be a problem for your child. Enough of the drug usually builds up in the child's system to protect against a single missed dose. And each dose is not large enough to cause a dangerously toxic blood level, although the child may be more drowsy or have an appetite change. If the missed dose is remembered within 48 hours, simply give it to the child in addition to regular doses. And if a double dose is given, don't skip any doses, just continue with the regular medication schedule.

However, repeatedly missing doses, or discontinuing the medication because the child hasn't had a seizure for a while, will almost certainly result in more seizures. Be honest with your doctor about how well the prescription has been followed. A blood test can be done to indicate if the child has been receiving the desired amount of medication. If you have problems getting your child to take the medication, ask your doctor or nurse for suggestions. Honesty and frankness between you and your health-care team will result in the best care for your child.

Even after seizures are under control, it may be necessary to change your child's medication program from time to time. Dosage may need to be increased or decreased, or a different medication used, to compensate for the child's growth, or because of changes in the epilepsy itself. This may become especially apparent as the child goes through puberty. Roughly 60% of children have fewer seizures after puberty, about 30% stay the same, and about 10% have more seizures.

CAN A CHILD WITH EPILEPSY TAKE OTHER KINDS OF MEDICATION?

In general, yes, but it is a good idea to avoid unnecessary nonprescription medications, such as cold remedies, because they seldom help the child and can interact with the antiepileptic medication. However, it is important for medical problems such as ear infections and asthma to be treated. To be safe, whenever a doctor prescribes a medication or immunization for the child, remind the doctor of the antiepileptic medication(s) the child is taking. Some prescription medications are known to interact with antiepileptic medications, and the doctor can prescribe something else. If you forget to ask the doctor, discuss this with the pharmacist.

IS IT EVER POSSIBLE TO DISCONTINUE A CHILD'S MEDICATION?

Yes it is, depending on the type of seizures the child had or is having. If there is a clear family pattern of having a certain type of seizures up until a certain age, that is a good guideline to follow in deciding when to try to discontinue a child's medication. If there is no family history to go on, but the child has been seizure-free for two to four years, it may be a good idea to gradually withdraw medications under the close supervision of the child's doctor. An EEG may be helpful in detecting whether the child is continuing to have abnormal brain electrical activity.

Also, if no cause was found for the child's seizures, and the child has been seizure-free for two years, it may be appropriate to taper the medication to find out if he still needs it. If a seizure occurs, the child should resume taking the medication and another attempt should be made two years later if he remains seizure-free. Anyone, at any age, who is taking antiepileptic medications and has been seizure-free for four years should probably make an attempt to reduce or discontinue medications. This should always be done with your doctor's consent and supervision.

WHAT IF MEDICATIONS DON'T CONTROL THE SEIZURES WITHOUT TOXICITY?

A small number of people with epilepsy have seizures that are very difficult to control. They may need to choose a treatment regimen that is somewhere between perfect seizure control and no toxicity. Again, though, don't be too quick to settle on an unacceptable medication unless all options have been exhausted. New antiepileptic medications are being tested in clinical research and approved by the Food and Drug Administration, so keep checking with your doctor or epilepsy center to see if a new medication might help your child.

Surgery is becoming an increasingly effective option for people whose seizures are not well controlled. A few seizures are still a few too many. This includes children, for whom certain types of surgery have proved to be safe and effective when performed in centers that have developed special expertise in epilepsy neurosurgery. If your child's seizures are not well controlled by medications, consider having the child evaluated at an epilepsy center to see if he or she is a candidate for surgery for epilepsy (see Chapter 8).

CAN A SPECIAL DIET SOMETIMES PREVENT SEIZURES?

A few children may benefit from a special diet to control seizures. Sometimes a diet high in fat will cause an imbalance in the child's body chemistry called ketosis. This sometimes results in better seizure control, but it is a difficult diet to follow. A similar dietary measure that has been successful in a few children is called a medium chain triglyceride (MCT) diet. It is more convenient than the ketogenic diet because it involves adding a special oil to the child's diet. Again, these dietary measures are helpful in only a small number of children with epilepsy. They should not be tried without a doctor's supervision, because they can be hazardous and lead to other health problems if not monitored closely.

The vast majority of children with epilepsy will benefit most from a healthy, well-balanced diet, possibly with the addition of a vitamin and mineral supplement. In fact, paying more attention to eating the right foods can help keep the whole family more healthy, with more energy to enjoy life and cope with its challenges. Ask your doctor or nurse about the best diet for your family.

WHAT SAFETY STEPS SHOULD BE TAKEN FOR A CHILD WITH EPILEPSY?

Part of the treatment of epilepsy is to make any necessary safety changes in the child's environment. Most children whose seizures are well controlled need very little if any special attention. However, all children need parents to exercise common sense on their behalf. For example, all children should be supervised when swimming or playing near water, and all children and adults should wear helmets when bicycling or skateboarding, because these activities result in thousands of head injuries every year. Likewise, appropriate safety equipment should be worn when participating in any sport or activity.

If a child's seizures are not well controlled, it may be necessary to take extra precautions, but it is best for children to have as much privacy and freedom as possible. For example, it may be wise to have someone present when a young child is bathing, because children have drowned in just inches of water after having a seizure. But as a child grows older he or she will naturally want privacy, so the supervision should be from an adjacent room. Also, for a younger child it is a good idea to remove locks from the bedroom, bathrooms, and any other area he has access to. A child with epilepsy should not sleep in the upper bunk of a bunkbed. And if he has seizures at night and falls out of bed, make sure that the floor is padded with carpeting or a rug. A medical ID bracelet is also a good idea, in case he is separated from parents. Ask your child's health-care team what other safety measures, if any, they recommend for your child.

WHAT TYPES OF ACTIVITIES ARE UNSAFE FOR A CHILD WITH EPILEPSY?

Most children with epilepsy can do pretty much everything other children can do. Any restrictions should be imposed only when warranted by the type of seizures a child has, not in an attempt to remove any and all sources of danger from the child's life. The following recommendations were developed by the American Académy of Pediatrics:

The responsibility for weighing the risks involved in athletic participation should be shared by the parents, the physician, and the child. Such risks should be weighed against the psychological trauma resulting from unnecessary restriction of physical activities. Parents should participate in all decisions. To the degree appropriate to the age and judgment of the child, his or her wishes should be considered. The young athlete must be taught that there is a risk of injury and he or she should be prepared to impose voluntary restrictions on physical activity depending upon the nature and frequency of seizures.

Proper medical management, good seizure control, and proper supervision are essential if children with epilepsy are to participate fully in physical education programs and interscholastic athletics. Common sense dictates that situations in which a seizure could cause a dangerous fall should be avoided. These situations include rope climbing, activity on parallel bars, and high diving. Swimming should be supervised; no competitive underwater swimming is acceptable. Participation in contact or collision sports should be given individual consideration according to the specific problem of the athlete. Epilepsy per se should not exclude a child from hockey, baseball, football, basketball, and wrestling.

Physicians who take care of children who are involved in athletics should realize that in today's culture, sports and athletic activity are extremely important to young people and that unnecessarily strict interpretation of medical conditions may in fact do more harm than good (*Pediatrics* 72:884–885, 1983).

Some children may have seizures more often when they are more active. This should be monitored and a strategy planned with the doctor to prevent the seizures, while allowing the child to be as active as possible. Medications may be timed to be most effective during periods in which he is most active. It may also help to make sure he gets more rest, eats more nutritious meals, and follows a consistent daily schedule in general. Many children and teenagers find that seizure control is much better with regular exercise.

Children who have seizures that cause them to fall can be allowed to participate in most activities, with perhaps a little more protective gear and supervision. They should not participate in climbing activities, however. Other activities in which a fall could be especially dangerous, such as horseback riding, may have to be prohibited.

Swimming is probably the most difficult activity for which to make recommendations. A child who has infrequent seizures can probably participate in swimming activities in which there is a buddy system, and in which a lifeguard supervises a small group of children. Wearing a lifejacket may provide an extra measure of protection, but it restricts the child's mobility in water activities. If a child will be allowed to go into the water, it is important that he receive swimming instruction in a certified teaching program. Swimming may be safe for children who experience occasional or frequent seizures, but only with close supervision in a restricted area, such as a pool or shallow, roped area of a lake.

When deciding which activities a child may participate in, emphasize the many things he can do, rather than the few things that are too dangerous. Help him develop strengths and obtain exercise and enjoyment from as many activities as possible. The next chapter suggests ways parents and others can help a child with epilepsy.

12

Helping a Child Live Well with Epilepsy

Judy L. Antonello, M.S.W., A.C.S.W.

Many factors are involved in helping a child live well with epilepsy. Proper diagnosis and treatment are certainly the first important steps. But as with all children, a child with epilepsy needs the love and support of parents who can help him enjoy life while meeting its challenges.

WHAT SPECIAL CHALLENGES ARE FACED BY PARENTS OF CHILDREN WITH EPILEPSY?

A major challenge for parents of a child with epilepsy is to help him grow up to be a self-confident adult—who just happens to have epilepsy. Often with chronic disorders that require daily treatment, parents with the best of intentions may focus on the child's disorder, so that he develops a self-concept that emphasizes the disorder. The child with epilepsy also soon realizes that other children don't have seizures, and the feeling of being different may lead to social isolation.

The risk of this happening can be reduced. Children with epilepsy can grow up to be active, self-assured, popular teenagers and adults. Epilepsy can be put in perspective in a loving and happy family environment. Professional help can be sought when there is uncertainty about how to handle things or just when an objective listener is needed. A balance can be achieved in the family life to help meet the new demands epilepsy brings and set the stage for the child to grow up a little more prepared to enjoy life and meet its challenges.

When a child is diagnosed with epilepsy, the family balance is almost always upset for a while. Naturally, everyone wants things to get back to where they were before. At first, parents and older brothers and sisters may go through a grieving process, in which each individual may feel a different swirling of emotions about the child and about epilepsy. Parents tend to have certain expectations and images about what a child's life will be like. Epilepsy may seem as if it has shattered these dreams. The family and those close to the family need to accept this grief as real and understandable.

Each family and each individual will proceed through the grieving process a little differently. Some may deny for a time that epilepsy exists. This helps some people gain the time they need to handle what has happened. It usually does not become a problem unless it interferes with the child's care or with family life, or if it persists for too long. Most people do progress through the various emotions to a point at which they can work toward accepting their child's epilepsy.

Changes can be made so the family can learn to cope with the new stress of epilepsy. What these changes are will depend on what type of treatment is necessary, and on how well controlled the child's seizures can be. Families adapt to these changes and stresses in different ways, some more quickly than others. If the family was experiencing problems before the diagnosis, it may be more difficult to handle the additional stress. Family members expressing feelings to each other and in professional counseling can help identify sources of family tension and assist the family in adapting and exploring alternatives.

Several things can be done to help reduce the stress that epilepsy can place on a family. All of these depend on good family communication, in which each family member feels welcome to share feelings and to contribute ideas.

First, it is important for everyone, children especially, to understand the situation as well as maturity allows (we'll discuss ways to explain epilepsy to children a bit later). Being open with children and helping them to understand epilepsy reduces their fear of the unknown, and lets them know what the reason is for the new tension they have probably detected in the family. If both parents are part of the family, each needs to be aware of and work toward understanding the diagnosis. Each should have a chance to ask questions of the health-care team. One parent may accept the main responsibility for overseeing the child's care, but it helps if both participate as much as possible.

Parents also can examine their own feelings about the child's epilepsy. It is natural to feel angry or resentful when a health problem disrupts an individual's and a family's life. Some parents feel guilty about this anger and have difficulty expressing it. This may lead to depression and sometimes to inappropriate expressions of anger. It may help for parents to discuss feelings such as anger with each other, friends, family, other parents of a child with epilepsy, or with a counselor, either individually or together.

When all family members have some understanding of epilepsy, the family can discuss any changes that will be helpful in daily life. This can be done in a matter-of-fact way that does not make it seem as if epilepsy will be a huge burden. Children need to know that epilepsy is serious, but they also need to be reassured that they can continue to enjoy many of the same interests as before, as well as new ones.

Some families greatly alter their lifestyle and routines in response to epilepsy. This can create resentment toward the child with epilepsy or toward the parent who is ordering all the changes. If there is a need to cut back on family outings or for family members to assume new responsibilities, it may help if everyone is involved in deciding how the changes will be made. By prioritizing which things are most important for family happiness, it is usually possible to identify ways of solving problems with a minimum of stress.

Another way to reduce stress on the family is to identify resources and increase sources of support both within and outside the family. Think of family balance as a seesaw, with stress on one end and support resources on the other. As stress is added to one end, it upsets the family balance. This balance can be restored by identifying and using sources of support and by seeking out community resources. These may include respite care, financial assistance, homemaker services, and home health services. Other valuable sources of support may include relatives, friends, and neighbors who may ask if they can help with child care, housework, or in other ways. Resources may include counselors, nurses, doctors, social workers, churches, government programs, epilepsy organizations, support groups for people with epilepsy and their families, and many other community programs (see Chapter 20). Finally, but most important, is the family becoming aware of what their own strengths really are.

Sometimes both or one of the parents of a child with epilepsy ignores their own interests and friends, believing that they need to attend more fully to the child's needs. Often this is because they have very little energy left for themselves. Parents' relationships with each other may be disrupted. Or the parent as a person may be temporarily lost. Parents who deny their own needs and goals in life can feel unfulfilled and depressed, which may leave them with less energy to care for their child. Happy children need happy parents. Taking care of oneself can allow for more energy to meet the demands that arise each day.

The opposite reaction to epilepsy may also occur, in which one or both parents throw themselves into interests outside of the home in an attempt to block out the pain of epilepsy. The parent may still be denying that the child has epilepsy. The other parent may have to take on more of the responsibility for taking care of the child with epilepsy, which may drain that parent's energy. Also, the child may feel the loss of the parent who is away and may even feel responsible.

Children readily detect withdrawal of a parent's attention and may perceive it as rejection. The child with epilepsy may believe that he or she is no longer loved because of epilepsy and may feel guilty for developing the disorder. Brothers and sisters may also feel responsible for the epilepsy, or they may resent their sibling for having it. Needless to say, these types of emotional fallout can be devastating to a family's health and happiness.

Sometimes parents or whole families can find themselves socially isolated after a child develops epilepsy. Friends may never call anymore or they may drift away. This is usually because of a lack of understanding about epilepsy, or because they just don't know what to say. It can help to take the initiative and call friends to tell them how you're doing. Explain the basics about epilepsy: that they can't catch it, that seizures are caused by a sudden uncontrolled burst of electricity in the brain, and that your child may have a seizure once in a while but is otherwise fine. Tell them that you value their friendship and don't want epilepsy to interfere with it. Most people will welcome such a conversation, because they may have been feeling guilty for avoiding you or feeling unsure about how to discuss epilepsy. With the air cleared, everyone can benefit from continuing friendships.

It may be difficult for parents and families to live well with the changes epilepsy brings. We've found that the families who do the best are the ones who:

- Openly discuss epilepsy and the changes that are needed
- Share their feelings with each other and with outsiders when they feel it may be helpful
- Make good use of support systems and resources
- Stay active as a family and as individuals in activities they enjoy
- Approach challenges confidently and optimistically, rather than reacting to problems with dismay and resignation.

HOW CAN PARENTS HELP THE CHILD WITH EPILEPSY DEVELOP A POSITIVE SELF-IMAGE?

Epilepsy poses some unique and difficult problems for children, because it is both an episodic and a chronic disorder. Seizures may occur unpredictably, affecting the child's sense of self-control as well as frustrating the parents' desire to protect him. Parents naturally must exercise a great deal of control over their children. But it helps to realize that children with epilepsy feel an added loss of control and can benefit from being allowed to make choices in certain areas of their lives.

A few additional controls are necessary because of epilepsy, such as making sure the child takes medications as prescribed. But parents may be too restrictive, such as not letting the child with epilepsy participate in relatively safe games with other children. This may reinforce the child's feeling of being different and lacking control over life. Children who are allowed to make the most out of their life while they are young tend to grow up with a healthy sense of control and a confidence that they can have a good life.

As they grow, children may attempt to find a sense of control through unwanted behaviors, such as being aggressive or demanding with family members and other children. If a child with epilepsy is feeling a lack of control, these behaviors may be extreme and persistent; the child may even learn to fake seizures to gain attention and control over others.

Parents have the large and often trying responsibility for steering children along a productive and happy course through the various stages of early development. Take advantage of your support system to give yourself a break when children become too much and threaten your self-control. This is not a sign of weakness, it is a sign of a parent who knows what is right for his or her children.

All children need to experience success and encouragement in order to develop a positive self-image. If a child with epilepsy is not given a chance to experience success and make decisions frequently in daily life, he may grow up feeling incapable of success and helpless to make any decisions or changes. The child may feel little responsibility for successes or failures, thinking that epilepsy, family, and society are in total control. Parents can help their child become aware of choices and encourage him to risk making decisions, which can lead to success and improved self-esteem. We've found the following suggestions to be helpful to some families.

Help your child achieve constructive control by providing choices rather than ultimatums whenever feasible. For example, rather than telling a child to put on a specific shirt, try asking him to choose from two or three. This gives the child experience with decision-making and gives him a sense of responsibility. Later, if someone comments on the shirt, the child can enjoy the feeling of responsibility for a successful decision. The reinforcement of many such successes will help the child to develop self-confidence and competence. A self-confident child is more likely to take the risk to make more decisions, starting a spiraling chain of increasing self-confidence, ability to handle responsibility, and self-esteem.

When a child refuses to obey, or refuses to make a choice among the alternatives offered by a parent, try helping him to see the consequences of not making a decision. For example, if given a choice of two chores to do and the child says "none," explain that if he doesn't decide which chore to do, he will have decided that a prediscussed consequence will result, such as not being able to watch a favorite television program. By pointing out a consequence of the child's decision, and by helping him see that he is deciding whether or not to enjoy the privilege, the parent is less likely to be singled out as the "bad guy."

For example, if the parent says, "You're deciding that you don't want to watch your favorite show," the child begins to realize that there are consequences to decisions and begins to feel a sense of responsibility. This will not take place overnight, of course, and it is not always possible to offer choices. But by giving the child such experience whenever possible, parents can help him develop a mature sense of responsibility.

Try to look beyond a child's behavior for the feelings behind it. Also try to help the child identify those feelings. This helps in three ways: it improves communication between child and parent, it lets the child know the parent cares about his or her feelings, and it helps the child be aware of feelings.

For example, your child comes home from school and begins slamming doors or throwing books on the floor. You can say, "You really seem mad right now. Do you want to talk about it?" He may or may not want to talk, but it lets him know that you are aware of and care about his feelings. If he does not want to talk, you may say, "That's fine, I just want you to know that I am here if you do want to talk about it." If the child does want to talk, it can help the parent understand what types of problems the child may be having, either because of epilepsy or from the normal difficulties of growing up.

It may be counterproductive to push the child to communicate. This can lead to a power struggle, in which the child gets attention as well as gaining control by denying the parent any access to feelings. But if he does want to talk about a problem, the parent can practice what is called "active listening." This involves listening carefully to how the child explains what happened, and then following it with a comment on what you think he was trying to tell you.

For example, if the child comes home and says another child was teasing him about epilepsy, the parent can respond with something like, "It sounds like you were pretty angry. What did you do?" Without criticizing the child's actions, ask him about other ways to respond. If he is blank, then offer a few alternatives to choose from. Do a little "brainstorming," helping the child to see possible consequences of each response. Rather than taking control of a fairly minor situation by calling the school or the other child's parents, or by telling the child to respond in a certain way, help him learn to handle life situations.

Follow up with the child to find out what action was taken and how it turned out. If there was a negative result, compliment him for trying and do some more brainstorming. If there was a positive result, compliment him and point out that it was his decision. If possible, generalize the situation to other problems the child may face, expressing confidence that he will be able to handle them equally well.

WHAT SHOULD BROTHERS AND SISTERS OF A CHILD WITH EPILEPSY BE TOLD ABOUT THE DISORDER?

Parents sometimes feel that they don't want to worry their children about a brother's or sister's epilepsy. But children often sense when something is being hidden from them. This can lead them to fill in missing information, and their imaginary details can be far worse than the truth. We encourage parents to be honest with their children.

It is important that parents sit down with children and explain epilepsy at a level they can understand. Put epilepsy into perspective by explaining that everyone has something that makes them different from other people. Wearing glasses, being left-handed, being short or tall, and many other things make people different. But different doesn't mean "bad." Explain that their brother or sister is just like everyone else, except that sometimes a little burst of electricity happens in the brain and a seizure occurs.

Also, explain that you may need to do some extra things with the child with epilepsy, such as going to the doctor or buying medication. Discuss any extra safety precautions that may be necessary. Tell the children what to do in case of a seizure, without putting more responsibility on a child than he or she can handle. Most children can understand that they need to remove any dangerous objects from the area and then tell an adult. As children grow older, make them aware of the first-aid steps in Chapter 9. Also, enlist them in the effort to educate others about epilepsy and in helping their brother or sister recover emotionally from a seizure.

It can be helpful to involve older brothers and sisters in caring for a child with epilepsy. There is a very real danger, however, of overburdening them. This can negatively affect their emotional and social development. We sometimes hear brothers or sisters says things like, "Not only do Mom and Dad spend all their time with (the child with epilepsy), they always make me take care of him too!"

A brother or sister may also become dedicated to caring for and protecting a sibling with epilepsy. They may somehow feel responsible for the epilepsy, or they may simply see this as the best way to gain attention and approval from their parents. This may create problems in the long run if the child becomes too worried about the sibling and limits outside social or recreational contacts.

Parents can cope with the possible problems involving siblings of a child with epilepsy by practicing the same type of communication and sharing of feelings that we discussed earlier. Ask children how they feel about epilepsy, or how they feel after their sibling has a seizure. Parents and children may feel very frustrated after a seizure, as if they should have been able to protect the child or prevent the seizure. It is important for everyone to remind each other that this is not possible.

It is fairly common for siblings to feel some embarrassment about the child with epilepsy. They may not want to bring friends home in case their brother or sister has a seizure. Parents must realize that this is a common feeling and not a reason to punish or chastise a child. It is another good time to practice communication skills. Make sure the child understands what a seizure is. Find out if he feels he can talk to his friends about his sibling's epilepsy. Help him figure out how to do this by explaining to his friends that epilepsy is not contagious, that it is not a sign of being crazy, and that they can't prevent seizures and don't need to be afraid if one should occur while they are visiting. Encourage him to have friends visit and let him know that you appreciate his understanding and love for his brother or sister.

Another problem we sometimes see is when parents treat a child with epilepsy differently than their other children. This is a common reaction, because parents often feel that the child with epilepsy has suffered enough in life and deserves special treatment. Some parents feel guilty that they may have caused the child's epilepsy by something they did wrong during pregnancy or while the child was an infant. If you are feeling somehow responsible for your child's epilepsy, it may help to discuss this with your doctor or with a counselor.

Giving special treatment to a child with epilepsy may increase his sense of being different. Children may take advantage of such special treatment to avoid responsibility and to gain attention and favors. It also gives them the message that they are different, because they are getting different attention than siblings or other children. This is not only unhealthy for the child with epilepsy, it can also cause resentment and anger from his brothers and sisters, hurting their relationship with the child with epilepsy and with their parents. It is possible to minimize these problems and build the child's self-esteem by adapting responsibilities to suit his abilities, while still having significant expectations.

Children benefit when parents recognize and encourage the wide range of good things they do, not just things like taking epilepsy medications or helping with the child with epilepsy. Both parents and children benefit when parents take time for themselves and for the other aspects of life. Spouses, friends, and relatives can help by being good listeners and letting the parent know you understand the feelings he or she is sharing.

HOW CAN I HELP MY CHILD WITH EPILEPSY MAKE FRIENDS?

Parents often are concerned that their child with epilepsy will have a more difficult time making friends. Children who have a reasonably good self-image will tend to attract friends. Parents can help build the child's confidence and self-esteem at home, and then he may develop more confidence in social situations away from home.

Some possible signs of problems may be if the child does not interact with others or seems withdrawn, shy, nervous, or anxious much of the time. He may avoid doing things other children are doing or may fight or cry when playing. Remember that all these things can be normal behavior. It is only if they become excessive or disruptive for the child that they indicate a possible problem.

Parents can help their child make friends by encouraging desirable social behavior and by praising appropriate behavior. Try encouraging social situations by allowing the child to choose a playmate to play a game with. This can be helpful at home or in a school or daycare situation. Ask the child if there is a friend who could be invited to come over and play. Involve him in appropriate organized activities to ensure there are plenty of chances to develop social skills and make friends. For an older child, try to avoid choosing his friends. Instead, encourage him to make friends and reinforce their socialization. As the child develops interests and strengths, continue by providing frequent opportunities in which he can enjoy socializing and experience success.

If you have younger children, you may want to try to meet parents with children the same age as yours. Discuss your interests and those of your child, and attempt to find out if your children might play well together. Epilepsy may enter this discussion, depending on how likely it is that your child may have a seizure while playing. Honesty is usually best, to prevent the possibility of surprise and fear for other parents if your child has a seizure at the other child's home. Again, provide some basic epilepsy facts to make sure the other parent has no misconceptions that would prevent your children from being friends. Give some simple first-aid tips and reassure them that they don't need to do anything to "treat" the seizure, and that they can call if the seizure continues. In fact, make sure they understand that it can be harmful to try to force anything into the child's mouth or to restrain him during a seizure. Thank them for understanding and for helping your child have a chance to develop socially.

Many parents find it helpful to include their child in telling others about epilepsy. Ask him how he would like it explained. Help the child learn to introduce the subject at an appropriate time, after a friend has gotten to know something about him as an individual.

As the child gets older, let him assume more of the responsibility for explaining epilepsy. This can help develop techniques for bringing epilepsy into conversations in a comfortable way and at an appropriate time. This skill will prove valuable when meeting people throughout life.

IS IT SAFE TO LEAVE A CHILD WITH EPILEPSY IN DAYCARE OR WITH A BABYSITTER?

Parents need occasional breaks from their children to be alone as individuals and as a couple. Children benefit from these breaks as well, because it helps them learn that they can survive and have a good time even when Mom and Dad are not there. Also, they benefit by returning to parents who are happier and more emotionally healthy.

Deciding on appropriate care for a child with epilepsy depends on how frequent his seizures are. If a child has rare or even occasional seizures, most daycare professionals will be able to care for him. Choose a daycare center or home setting carefully, as you would for any child. Talk with parents who now have or have had their children in the setting and visit the daycare location during the day to see what types of activities children are involved in. Some states certify daycare providers after inspection of the setting. If your state does not certify centers, be as thorough in checking the safety of the daycare environment as you are with your own home. Inform prospective care providers about your child's epilepsy, and discuss how comfortable they would feel dealing with seizures.

After selecting a daycare provider, discuss your child's medical care with all daycare staff. Make sure they know when and how to give his medication. Inform them about the type of seizures he experiences and discuss the first-aid steps necessary. Tell them when you would like to be informed of a seizure, and discuss when it might be necessary to call for emergency assistance if the child's seizures last longer than usual or if he is hurt.

Discuss the reason for daycare with your child in a manner suited to the child's ability to understand. Make sure the child knows that you will be returning and that you are confident that he or she will have fun. As he gains experience in daycare, ask open-ended questions to try to get as much information as possible about feelings and activities during the day. Be open with the care provider about your child's needs, fears, and problems. Provide suggestions without appearing harshly critical. And don't forget to provide positive feedback and express appreciation whenever appropriate. A good relationship with the daycare provider makes everyone's days go smoother.

A child with occasional seizures can also be left safely with a mature teenager or adult. Check the sitter's references and discuss the child's seizures and first aid at a get-acquainted session before needing the sitter's services. Give the child a chance to get to know the sitter while you are still there, and provide a detailed outline for the sitter to follow when you are gone. Make sure the sitter understands the first-aid instructions and knows when to call you and when it might be necessary to call the emergency number. If the sitter will be giving the child medication, remind her that the child must get the full dose, and that, if there is any spillage or any is spit out, to have the child take that portion again. Check with the sitter as often as you feel the need, but remember that you need to take advantage of the time to relax and enjoy yourself.

If a child has many seizures during the day, parents will be in even greater need of time to rest and enjoy outside activities. Friends or relatives can usually be taught to care for a child with frequent seizures. Other options exist in most communities, such as health-care centers where trained nurses provide care to handicapped children, or people who provide in-home or out-of-home care known as "respite care." This type of care is available through many county human service agencies. The fee is usually adjusted according to a family's income. Respite care is often provided by licensed people or, when medically necessary, by nurses.

HOW CAN PARENTS HELP THEIR CHILD WITH EPILEPSY GET THE MOST OUT OF SCHOOL?

Under a federal law passed in 1975 and known as the Education of All Handicapped Children Act (Public Law 94-192), public and private schools must provide an adequate education to all children, regardless of handicap. Schools must allow a handicapped child to participate in regular classrooms as long as he is able to benefit from that experience more than from an education in a specially adapted program. This is sometimes difficult to judge, but most children with epilepsy can participate fully in regular classrooms.

Most schools are willing to do whatever they can to help a child with epilepsy. Parents can help them by meeting with the school nurse and with the child's teacher each year, and with administrators as necessary. Discuss your child's seizures and treatment program, as well as your perceptions about how he is dealing with epilepsy. Make sure the teacher understands first aid for seizures and is aware of any learning difficulties your child may have. Suggest strategies that were useful in past school experiences, and encourage the teacher to talk with your child's previous teacher. For your child to get the most out of the school experience, it is very important that the teacher feels informed about and comfortable with his epilepsy. A letter from the child's doctor about his capabilities, restrictions if any, and medical needs may be reassuring.

Parents can also suggest ways the teacher can discuss epilepsy with the child's classmates. The school and the teacher should be aware of his epilepsy even if seizures occur very rarely. This avoids the danger and anger that might result from a seizure occurring with no preparation. If it is likely that the child will have a seizure in class, it is best to discuss epilepsy and seizures before one occurs. The child can often be involved in doing a little presentation for the class, with the teacher's help. Epilepsy can be placed in context with other disorders that affect some children, such as diabetes and cystic fibrosis. If a seizure occurs at school, a major factor in how other children will react is how calmly the teacher handles the situation.

Probably the most devastating thing that can happen to a child is to have a seizure that involves convulsions and loss of urinary or bowel control in front of a large group of peers. We have found that recovery from this experience depends largely on how the teacher discusses it with classmates. Parents can help by suggesting appropriate ways for the teacher to explain epilepsy to different age groups.

For example, preschoolers will be very open in asking questions about what they have observed. During the seizure the teacher can reassure the children that "Tommy" will be okay. The teacher can suggest a way they can occupy themselves while the child having the seizure is being cared for. Afterward, the teacher can explain that Tommy's brain told him to have a seizure, but he's okay now. The children can be told that they are not going to have a seizure, that they can't catch it from Tommy, and that they did not do anything to cause it. They should know that Tommy may have another seizure some time, but that he can play with them just like before and they need not worry about the seizure. Children should be encouraged to ask any questions they may have, and the teacher can involve Tommy in discussing seizures if the parents think this is appropriate. The important thing with preschoolers is to dispel any fear they may have about the seizure.

With elementary school children, teachers can use slides and movies to provide education about epilepsy. At this age, children are most concerned about safety for themselves and classmates. They may want to know if "Tommy" can control when a seizure occurs. They may also have some fear about epilepsy and whether or not they might develop the disorder. The teacher can explain that epilepsy means a person has seizures, which are caused by the brain sending the wrong message. Different types of seizures can be discussed. If appropriate, the child can explain his or her epilepsy and discuss how it feels to have a seizure. At this age, the main objective is to provide accurate information to head off any false ideas or ridicule that might result from a seizure.

In high school, a teacher can use verbal instruction to inform students about epilepsy. Students will be better able to generalize from their classmate's seizure to a health disorder affecting large numbers of people. They can benefit more from a discussion of how the brain works, and how the electrical activity in the brain can develop an abnormal pattern that results in a seizure. Their concern usually focuses less on safety and more on what they can do to help. At this age, it can be especially effective for the student with epilepsy to do a written or oral report on epilepsy, and to lead or participate in a class discussion of chronic health disorders. The important thing for a high school teacher is to build a positive attitude among classmates, so that if a seizure does occur they are more likely to want to do something for their classmate rather than resort to ridicule or aversion.

Of course, there will always be some children and adults who will bully or ridicule others. The child with epilepsy—and his classmates—need to understand that they can't control such people. But they can control how they feel about themselves and about each other. If the child with epilepsy is confident and asserts that the people who ridicule others are the ones with the real problem, peers and teachers will admire that strength of character.

Children with epilepsy benefit most when a school and teachers create an attitude of acceptance and understanding. This includes giving the child equal access to school resources. While the intellectual abilities of most children with epilepsy fall within the normal range, some may have minor or major learning delays or disabilities. It is crucial for the child's education that any delays or disabilities be discovered early and assessed accurately. Denial of or overemphasis on a child's deficit are both harmful. Insisting that a child with learning delays or disabilities attend regular classes with no special help can frustrate the child and prevent advancement. Likewise, pulling a child with learning difficulties out of all regular interaction with peers can severely damage social learning and self-esteem.

The Epilepsy Foundation of America (EFA) sponsors a program called Epilepsy School Alert. Packets of informational materials are available for teachers (their role in helping the student with epilepsy, hidden signs of epilepsy-related problems, and first-aid steps) and more general information for their students. Many local EFA affiliates will send a representative to a school with audiovisual materials to speak with teachers and students.

Parents need to work with the child's school to assess his intellectual abilities and place him in the best learning environment. Consultation with a child psychologist or psychiatrist, or with a childhood-learning specialist, may provide parents and the school with an objective opinion of what is best for the child.

Children with epilepsy are best served when their parents cooperate with the school. However, if the school refuses to include the child in activities for which he or she is qualified, parents may need to seek outside help. Most epilepsy programs or local EFA affiliates can refer parents to a disability advocate, a person trained to help people stand up for their own rights or for their child's. The advocate provides information and may accompany parents to meetings with school officials at which the child's situation and legal rights can be discussed. The advocate can also help parents decide when the assistance of a lawyer may be necessary, although this should be considered a last resort.

IS IT SAFE FOR A CHILD WITH EPILEPSY TO GO AWAY TO CAMP?

Many parents feel that they can't trust anyone to care for their child for any length of time, such as a one-week or two-week camp experience. This is a hard thing for any parent, but having this experience is a good rehearsal of the "letting go" that will happen as a child becomes an adult.

It is usually safe—and very beneficial—for children with epilepsy to attend a camp. What type of camp depends on the child's interests, skills, and seizure control. There are camps for children with epilepsy (see Chapter 20), but for most children this should not exclude consideration of other camps. Discuss the choice of a camp with your child's health-care team to help decide whether concerns about epilepsy may restrict your choice of a camp. It may be possible for your child to attend any type of camp, with restrictions on just a few activities, as discussed in the previous section.

To help you and your child become more comfortable with a particular camp, visit the camp and talk with the staff to develop some trust in their ability to take care of your child. Most camps have a family day, at which you could talk with some of the children and their parents to see how they feel about the camp. This visit will introduce your child to the camp environment and will alleviate fear of the unknown.

If you decide that you would feel comfortable with your child attending the camp, discuss it in an encouraging way with your child. Let your child know that you will miss him or her, but that you trust the camp staff and the child's ability to take care of things. Discuss any fears or anxiety your child may have, stressing that these are normal feelings. Help the child look forward to all the fun at camp and to meeting new friends.

The camp experience is a major step in building a child's self-esteem and confidence. It provides the child with the opportunity for more socialization and with the chance to gain confidence in his or her own self-reliance. These opportunities can increase the child's self-esteem and lead to even more social confidence. And the more the parent sees the child as competent and confident, the easier it is to let go in situations the child will encounter as an adolescent and young adult.

13

Transition to Independence:
Epilepsy in the Teen Years

Robert J. Gumnit, M.D., and Judy L. Antonello, M.S.W., A.C.S.W.

Adolescence is a time of extremes: happiness and sadness, excitement and anger, love and hate. The emotions and events of the teen years make them the most memorable times of most people's lives. Because of them, adolescence is seldom an easy time for teenagers or those close to them. Adolescence is the time when a young person begins to feel the need to make decisions and take action independently of parents. Mistakes will be made by all, but that is not necessarily bad—as long as we learn from them.

Probably the one factor that can contribute most to a positive adolescence is an ability and feeling of freedom to communicate. This doesn't mean forced parent–teen conferences; it means an atmosphere in which concerns can be discussed openly with parents, friends, and one or more other adults close to the teenager. In this atmosphere, boundaries can be set for both the teenager and parents through mutual discussion of the reasons for those limits.

Adolescence is a crucial time in anyone's life, but it can be particularly difficult for the teenager with epilepsy or any other chronic disorder or handicap. This is a time when one develops the self-concept and coping abilities to live in a world designed primarily for people without medical disorders. Epilepsy is an additional stress on this transition to independence. The teenager doesn't look any different from his friends but is aware of a difference and often emotionally exaggerates it. As an added reminder of this difference, the teenager with epilepsy sometimes is not allowed to do what his peers are doing.

There are no easy answers for these problems, but this chapter provides some suggestions for making adolescence a more enjoyable time of growth and change. We hope that both parents and teenagers will use this chapter as a common ground for learning from each other.

HOW DOES EPILEPSY AFFECT A TEENAGER'S ABILITY TO LIVE A NORMAL LIFE AND BECOME AN INDEPENDENT ADULT?

Probably the best way to describe the effect of epilepsy on teenagers and their parents is to say that it further confuses matters. Think of all the changes that occur as a young person enters puberty, begins dating, experiences the highs and lows of high school, and then makes decisions about further schooling and occupation. Many factors enter into how the teenager copes with each challenge, temptation, and frustration. Most teenagers and parents find themselves bewildered at times by this process. It is hard enough to try to understand the hormonal and psychological roller coaster of adolescence without the added confusion seizures may bring.

A family's response to the teen years will depend greatly on how they set limits and settled problems during childhood (see the previous chapter). If a pattern of open communication and positive reinforcement has been established, the family will be less likely to react with silence and distrust during this period. Crises may still occur, but they will probably not result in dangerous rifts that can cut off the teenager's receptiveness to parental love and guidance.

Parents who have the healthiest relationships with their teenagers tend to be those who feel it is their responsibility to help the child mature into an adult who is as independent as possible. Parents whose children have the most trouble becoming independent seem to be those who feel that their major responsibility is to protect the child from harm.

Parents should set realistic limits to protect their children, while realizing that every child will encounter risks in life. It is not beneficial to shield children from every possible danger, embarrassment, or chance of failure. To do so would deny their children the right to learn to face the world independently. Children raised in this way will enter adolescence knowing that they can rely on their parents for guidance and support, but that they must make their own decisions. They experience failure as well as success, and learn to feel responsible—and proud of—the outcomes of their actions.

A health disorder such as epilepsy puts even more emphasis on the parents' approach to the job of parenting. If the parents control all medical decisions and prevent the teenager from taking any social or physical risks, it is less likely that he will have a chance to mature into an independent adult. But if parents gradually let the teenager take responsibility for medications and health care, and set reasonable limits within which he can explore and enjoy the world, he will most likely have an enriching adolescence and become a self-confident, independent adult.

IS IT POSSIBLE FOR A TEENAGER TO OUTGROW EPILEPSY?

It is possible to outgrow epilepsy, and many people have fewer or less severe seizures as they become adults. Unfortunately, doctors are not yet able to tell who will have fewer problems with epilepsy as they get older. The exception to this is absence seizures, which are usually outgrown in adolescence or young adulthood.

It is also possible that seizures will become more frequent and more severe during adolescence, as the hormonal changes and growth spurts that occur during adolescence affect the way the body metabolizes medications. This can usually be controlled with changes in medication. It may be necessary to schedule more frequent visits to the doctor during the teen years, and to have blood level tests more often.

While there is no guarantee that a person will outgrow epilepsy, there is no reason not to hope that this will happen.

IS IT A GOOD IDEA TO KEEP EPILEPSY A SECRET FROM OTHERS?

Secrecy used to be the preferred approach with epilepsy, because there was a great deal of public fear and official discrimination toward those with the disorder. But as doctors became more knowledgeable about epilepsy and as families and organizations worked to win rights for those with the disorder, public and official attitudes have begun to change. There is still too much public misunderstanding, but that is partly because not enough people are willing to talk openly about epilepsy and to educate others.

Secrecy not only prevents public understanding, but also contributes to a negative self-image. A teenager who is told to hide something about himself is probably going to feel guilty or ashamed. This may lead to avoiding others for fear of being found out. A better approach is to consider epilepsy as just one way a person can be different. Epilepsy is an unfortunate difference, but one that is shared by others, many of whom have overcome it to lead active, happy lives.

The decision about who and when to tell should be arrived at mutually by the teenager and parents. The right of every individual to privacy must be weighed against a bad decision based on fear and ignorance.

Each person must decide how to tell others about epilepsy. School officials, teachers, and coaches should definitely be told, and the parents and teenager should meet with them to discuss how medications and seizures should be handled. Some teenagers will show no effects from medications and may never have a seizure at school. Others may have good and bad days. Teachers should know what to expect in order to help the teenager get the most out of the high school experience.

It is also a good idea for the teenager to tell friends with whom he or she spends a good deal of time. They should know what type of seizure their friend may have and what to do in case one occurs. These friends should also know whether or not the teenager wants them to tell others that he or she has epilepsy.

When and what to tell other peers usually depends on how often seizures occur. If seizures occur rarely or not at all during the day, a person may decide to tell only close friends. This prevents others from judging him or her based on prior beliefs about epilepsy. As a teenager makes new friends, they can be told in a way that lets them know they have nothing to fear but much to offer in the way of understanding and support. This type of sharing of personal information can increase the bond between two teenagers of either the same or opposite sex.

If frequent seizures occur at school, the best policy is probably to be open about discussing epilepsy in classes and with anyone who asks. This will dispel misunderstandings about the disorder and reduce the tendency of teenagers to ridicule those who are different. In fact, most teenagers will feel empathy for a peer confronted with a chronic health disorder. If they see that the person handles epilepsy confidently and with courage, they will probably admire him.

Of course, there will always be those who will make fun of or be mean to a person who has seizures or any other visible difference. There is little that can be done about this, except to realize that they are not the type of people you would want to be friends with anyway. The best way to discourage their taunts is to try not to be visibly upset by them. It may even help to think of and rehearse clever responses with friends or parents. Again, if others see that a bully's teasing has little effect or backfires, they will tend to side with the person being teased, which will further discourage the bully. If such actions become violent, a teenager needs to feel confident that school officials will be helpful. If not, the parents should become involved and help the school decide how to prevent further problems.

HOW SHOULD I HANDLE THE SUBJECT OF EPILEPSY WHEN DATING?

This depends largely on how comfortable you feel talking about your epilepsy. Everyone gets nervous when they begin dating, and there is no reason to make yourself more nervous by talking about epilepsy before you are ready. It may be better at first to date someone who already knows you have epilepsy. If this is not possible, consider whether your date needs to know about your epilepsy for safety reasons. If not, wait until you are comfortable with each other, and then bring the subject up the same way you did with your friends of the same sex.

Here are several tips about dating that teens with epilepsy have shared with us:

1. When first dating someone, arrange a group date. This makes conversation easier and helps everyone get to know each other without the pressure of being alone.

2. Before asking someone on a date, or when trying to attract the interest of someone, try to get to know him or her better at school. Talk to him in class or whenever you have a chance. After a few conversations his reaction will give you a good idea whether or not he would be willing to date you.

3. Find out what the other person likes to do and then suggest it as something you could do together. This can work as well for girls as for boys. Many boys will be too shy to ask a girl out even if they like her. But if a girl is friendly and begins discussing an activity, the boy may be encouraged to ask her out, or she can ask him out.

4. If a boy or girl turns down your request for a date, don't give up. He or she may just want to get to know you better before dating. If he or she starts avoiding you, turn your attention to someone else. Everyone experiences rejection at some time in his life. But if you continue to be friendly toward other people, you will find that there will always be someone who wants to get to know you better.

5. If you have trouble making conversation, arrange to do something active when first dating someone. Activities such as bowling or tennis are better than going out to eat, where you will be alone with the other person and will feel more pressure to think of things to talk about.

6. Remember that dating is supposed to be enjoyable—don't put so much pressure on yourself that you turn it into a tense, exhausting experience. This can happen if you worry too much about how to act to impress the other person, or whether or not to kiss or "make out." For some reason, one of the hardest things to do when first dating someone is to "act like yourself." But the more you can relax and let things happen naturally, the more you will enjoy dating. It is natural to want to engage in kissing and other intimate sharing. Let these things come gradually, as you become more comfortable with each other. Talk about your feelings and find out what the other person is comfortable with before you attempt to become more intimate.

DOES EPILEPSY AFFECT DEVELOPMENT OR EXPRESSION OF SEXUALITY?

In general, teenagers with epilepsy grow and develop just like anyone else. Some antiepileptic medications may reduce sexual feelings if the dosage is too high. But epilepsy does not prevent people from feeling and expressing normal sexual emotions.

It is important to realize that there is a wide range of "normal" sexual feelings, and a wide age range during which these feelings begin. If you have concerns or questions about your sexuality, find someone knowledgeable to talk to. This may be a parent or other relative, your doctor, a teacher, or a counselor.

Teens must make many decisions about sexuality—how, when, why, and with whom to express these feelings and experience intimate behavior. Friends are the most frequent source of communication about these decisions. This sharing of feelings and information is important and can be helpful. But it can also be misleading, because even friends tend to exaggerate or bend the truth when talking about sex. Parents and other adults can be another source of information and advice, but some adults are not comfortable talking about sex with their own teenagers or with other teens. If you find that an adult is not being helpful or seems to be uncomfortable talking with you, ask your doctor or school counselor to recommend someone you can talk with. This may be the most important and mature step you can take in developing your own sexuality.

HOW CAN TEENS AND PARENTS DEAL WITH REBELLIOUS BEHAVIOR?

Part of becoming independent is having strong ideas of your own and wanting to make your own decisions about how you behave. Therefore, every teen is likely to argue with or disobey a parent at some time, no matter what type of parent–child relationship has been developed. There may also be times of open rebellion, and these can be the toughest tests of a parent's patience and love. These are the times when teens most need their parents' help and support.

When a teenager has a health disorder such as diabetes or epilepsy, it is common for the disorder to become a focus of rebellion. Many teens will deny that they have the disorder or insist that it is going to go away soon. They may refuse to take medications or deliberately do things that will cause a seizure. Parents can help by gently helping the teen see the consequences of skipping medications. Keep making statements such as, "I'm proud that you continue to hope that your epilepsy will go away or be cured, because I feel the same way. We're not going to give up and let it take over our lives, like it would if you stopped taking your medications."

If a seizure occurs because medications were skipped, don't dwell too much on the seizure or the fact that it could have been prevented. Focus instead on the future, expressing confidence that the teenager will want to be as healthy and active as possible. Continue to help him remember to take medications, get enough rest, and eat properly, but make it clear that these are his own responsibilities. Remind the teenager that the reward for these actions is feeling good and being able to do the things that are important in his or her life—such as driving a car!

HOW DO ALCOHOL AND ILLEGAL DRUGS AFFECT EPILEPSY?

There is no way of determining how the use of alcohol or illegal drugs will affect a person's epilepsy. Some people can drink small or moderate amounts of alcohol without increasing seizure frequency. However, frequent drinking often leads to lack of sleep and poor nutrition, which can cause a person to have a seizure. And very heavy drinking is very likely to cause a seizure in most people with epilepsy, as well as in some who do not have epilepsy. Teenagers cannot drink legally in most states, so arrest and legal penalties must be considered as possible effects of alcohol on teenagers. And, finally, driving after drinking or riding in a car with someone who has been drinking is a leading killer in this country.

Illegal drugs vary so much in content and potency that it is difficult to predict the effect of any one drug or any one experience. The only thing for sure is that there is a great deal of danger in taking illegal drugs. Any substance intended to alter one's body or mind has certain inherent dangers. Even legal medications can be dangerous, which is why they are so strictly regulated. With illegal drugs, there is no regulation, and it is often to the seller's advantage to tamper with the contents of a drug. You may think you are "just" smoking a little marijuana or snorting cocaine, when in reality you are exposing yourself to contaminated chemicals mixed in disease-carrying containers. And sharing needles for injecting drugs is the second-leading cause of the spread of AIDS, after sexual intercourse. There is no way anyone can know what the chances are that taking a drug will make you high, make you have a seizure, make you very sick, or even make you dead.

Serious risks exist even if the drug you take is exactly what you have been told it is. Most illegal drugs affect the brain, which is where seizures originate. Therefore, the effect of a drug is likely to be a double whammy on the part of the brain affected by epilepsy, greatly increasing the chance of a seizure. Also, illegal drugs—especially uppers and downers—can be extremely dangerous when mixed with antiepileptic medications.

One of the most important decisions a teenager must make is whether or not to go along with peers who are breaking the law by drinking alcohol or taking illegal drugs. There is no doubt of the potential damage alcohol and drugs can cause. But there is also no denying that some people will survive repeated drunken or drug-induced experiences without becoming addicted or suffering other consequences. Each person must consider what he or she wants to achieve in life, and then consider whether it is worth risking the physical, emotional, and social dangers involved with the illegal use of alcohol or drugs.

CAN PEOPLE WITH EPILEPSY GET A DRIVER'S LICENSE?

Yes, but most states require that an applicant provide a doctor's statement that he or she has not had a seizure for a certain period of time—usually from six months to a year. Most states also require the doctor or driver to report any seizures and to provide a note each year stating that the driver is still seizure-free. See Chapter 19 for more information.

Teenagers and adults can often take part of the driver's training lessons even if they have not been seizure-free for the required period of time. Then, if their seizures are controlled, they will be ready to take the driving test.

The right to drive can be a powerful incentive to take medications on schedule and to do whatever else is necessary to prevent seizures. If you are not happy with your current seizure control, ask your doctor if there is anything else you can try. Or you may want to see a neurologist or visit an epilepsy center to get help in improving your seizure control.

Not being able to drive can make life difficult, but it does not prevent a determined person from being socially active, holding a job, and enjoying life. Many people with epilepsy have learned to enjoy riding the bus, have joined a carpool, or have friends who can drive them places. One man with epilepsy we know put it this way: "No one can tell me that I should learn to make the best of it—I had to decide that for myself. And I'm still hoping that I can go seizure-free long enough to get my license."

WHAT TYPE OF SPORTS ARE SAFE FOR A PERSON WITH EPILEPSY?

Most sports and activities are as safe for a person with epilepsy as they are for anyone else. Rather than ruling out any sports, it is best to consider interests, abilities, and medical condition before deciding if participation in a specific sport is wise.

If a teenager has frequent seizures without warning, it is a good idea to avoid any activity that is performed above the ground, in the water, or on hard surfaces. For example, riding a bicycle, swimming, and gymnastics would not be advisable. But wrestling, cross-country skiing, and track-and-field sports might be suitable.

If a teenager's seizures are fairly well controlled, there are few restrictions in terms of sports. The coaches and monitors should be informed that the person has epilepsy and should know proper first aid. When swimming, a buddy should always be within reach, and you should stay in an area with a lifeguard. And in all sports and activities, teenagers with epilepsy should have the benefit of the proper safety equipment, as should anyone participating in sports.

HOW CAN I PLAN FOR A CAREER OR JOB, NOT KNOWING HOW EPILEPSY WILL AFFECT MY ABILITY TO SUCCEED?

The most important part of anyone's preparation for a successful occupation is education. Your first goal should be to graduate from high school and get the most you can out of that experience. The interests and aptitudes you develop in high school will guide you toward occupations you might want to consider. Ask for help from your high school guidance counselor in preparing yourself as much as possible for those types of work.

After you leave high school it will probably become more apparent how much—if at all—your epilepsy will affect your ability to get a job, pursue vocational training, or go to college. Don't rule out any one of these options before discussing it with your guidance counselor, a job training counselor from the EFA's TAPS program, and your doctor. (See Chapter 17 for more information on employment training and placement.)

Getting a job can be a major step in the transition from adolescence to adulthood. There are people with epilepsy in almost every occupation you can think of—doctors, bankers, clerks, athletes, cabinetmakers, janitors, scientists, and teachers. Epilepsy may throw some tough challenges and frustrating setbacks your way. But, by setting your sights on a few realistic goals and taking the steps needed to achieve them, you can succeed as an independent adult. In the next chapter we'll discuss how successful adults solve problems and reach goals.

14

The Successful Adult with Epilepsy

Doug G. Heck, Ph.D.

This chapter will encourage you to think about your goals in life and your personal definition of success. It discusses the social and psychological problems that people with epilepsy sometimes face and describes how those problems can be dealt with and overcome.

IS IT POSSIBLE FOR AN ADULT WITH EPILEPSY TO BE SUCCESSFUL?

That may seem like a silly question, but many people think that having a chronic health problem makes it almost impossible to live a happy and productive life. They focus only on the problems that can be caused by diabetes, arthritis, or epilepsy, and are probably unaware of the thousands of people who refuse to let these problems prevent them from doing the things they realistically can.

Successful people have many things in common, but perhaps the most important factors are a clear idea of things they *can* achieve and a step-by-step plan for achieving them. This plan might not be formally written out on paper. It might just be a pattern of behavior—a way of setting a goal and then taking one step at a time to achieve that goal.

However, you may find it helpful to write out your plan in as much detail as you can. Start by deciding on a goal you want to achieve. Make sure it is realistic and takes into account those things in your life that can't be changed, while focusing on things that you *can* change. Then think of several small steps that will lead to this goal.

For example, if getting a job is your goal, you will first want to find out what type of work you are qualified for. Your first step might be to meet with an employment counselor to get advice about what types of jobs you do and how to apply for them. Or you may want to get some kind of training for a certain type of job. Then, you could make out a list of appropriate companies, using the want ads, the yellow pages, or the state or county employment service. Your next step could be to make a schedule to apply at one or two companies each day or week, whatever works into your schedule. When you first write your plan you will want to include a reminder that it is unlikely that you will be hired by the first company you visit.

Trying to take steps that are too big (such as applying for a job before getting the training or education it requires) often leads to discouragement. Instead, plan small steps that you can achieve with a reasonable amount of effort.

When designing your plan, be realistic about the problems that may occur, and plan how to deal with them. Everyone has setbacks and temporary failures. Successful people do two things to recover: they remind themselves that no one is perfect and everyone has problems, and they reward themselves for trying. Of course, it is important not to choose rewards that would add to the problem (for example, if your goal is to lose 20 pounds, you don't want to reward yourself for losing 5 pounds by eating a whole pizza!). Choose rewards that you can afford and that you enjoy— things like going to a movie.

While designing your plan, practice giving yourself positive messages about each step. For example, if you are going to apply for a job and the first person turns you down, you may tell yourself, "I knew this wasn't going to be easy. I have to go on to the next interview, remembering the tips I read about (Chapter 17), and acting like the cheerful, hard-working, competent person I really am." Also, think about any negative messages you may unconsciously be giving yourself. Thoughts like "I am starting to have more seizures now, so my life is probably going down the drain" can lead to generalizations, such as "I'll never succeed at anything, because I have epilepsy." These messages are not only inaccurate, but they seriously affect the way you approach challenges. By substituting a message such as "I may have epilepsy, but I'm a hard worker who doesn't give up easily," you not only help yourself, you convince others that you can help them.

Most of all, have fun designing your plan! Life doesn't turn out to be fun by accident; each of us has to make it that way. By taking time to carefully plan for success, you will force yourself to reflect on what you want to change and what you want to achieve. When done with enthusiasm and hope, this planning can be fun. It can help you identify your strengths and weaknesses. Rely heavily on your strengths when designing your plan, but don't forget to laugh at yourself and at life now and then. If you encounter a person who is unpleasant, or if you experience a situation that turns out badly, repeat your positive messages to yourself. Give yourself credit for trying and for surviving a tough situation, which everyone faces now and then. By analyzing the situation and learning from it, you will be better prepared for the next attempt to achieve an important step on the way to your goal.

Let's look at one example of a plan, one in which the goal is to obtain a job that you feel good about and enjoy.

Step 1: Determine Your Interests

A good initial step is to determine what type of work you are interested in doing. Do you enjoy working with people or do you prefer working alone? Indoors or outside? Physical labor or more along the line of clerical work? Seek out information on types of jobs through your local library or state job and training office. Consider types of work in which you may have already gained some experience. A job counselor can help you become more aware of your interests through specialized testing.

Step 2: Determine Your Abilities

It is important to carefully match the type of work you are seeking with your capabilities. Most people can identify characteristics about themselves that will be helpful in a job setting, such as being able to communicate well with others. However, most people also experience things that are more difficult. For example, some people who have epilepsy may have a difficult time with their memory. In this case, it would be important to look for a type of work that does not require a lot of remembering, or one that would allow you to write down information as needed. Again, specialized testing through a job counselor may be especially useful in determining your strengths and how to match them to a type of job.

Step 3: Develop Prevocational Skills

In this step, it is important to become knowledgeable and trained in the many different areas that will assist you in finding a job and keeping it. For example, it is wise to learn about the process of applying for a job, how to interview as well as possible, and to know how or when to disclose your epilepsy to a potential employer. It may also be helpful to improve your communication skills, assertiveness, listening skills, and the actual skills needed for the job you desire. This may involve taking classes, or working in a training program or with various professionals. Building up your skills through volunteer work can also be helpful.

Step 4: Apply for Jobs

This is the step in which you actually try for the type of job you've identified as one that you are prepared for and interested in, using the skills you've developed.

Other personal goals for which you could prepare a plan might include: Develop better relationships with specific others. Or become more active socially. The actual goals you set for yourself will depend on your own set of values and your personal definition of success.

After designing your plan, be sure to make an honest attempt to follow it through. For example, if your goal is to get a job, and the first step is to seek occupational counseling, don't put off making an appointment. *You* are the only judge of how hard you have tried. If you repeatedly fail at the first step, perhaps it is too big a step. Try to break it down even further into more manageable achievements. As long as you keep trying, you haven't failed. Make sure to take one step at a time.

Deal with problems and setbacks according to plan. Reward yourself for trying, not just for succeeding. And when you do succeed, build that success into your self-messages. Then go on to try the next step. That's probably the most meaningful definition of a successful adult: one who keeps taking the next step to achieve a goal.

HOW CAN I MOTIVATE MYSELF TO CONTROL EPILEPSY AND ACHIEVE MY GOALS?

First of all, it is important to realize that no one is motivated all the time. It is normal for motivation to wax and wane. You may feel more motivated when you are most healthy, perhaps because you have been sleeping well, eating the right foods, taking your medications as scheduled, and things are going well. You may feel least motivated when you're tired and nothing seems to be going right, which leads you to eat poorly and perhaps forget your medication. There will be times when you don't have the energy to change your life. But this is normal.

Take advantage of times when you feel well, and do your best to help yourself feel well. Think of what you need to do to follow a healthy lifestyle, not just because that is best for your body, but because it is usually directly related to your state of mind, and to feeling motivated. Use those times when you feel most motivated to design your plan, and then do your best to carry it out.

If you feel that in general you are not motivated to try to achieve anything, it is important to find the reason why. First, it's important to see if your medication may be responsible for making you feel tired or depressed. Be sure to discuss this with your physician. Then consider whether you are depressed, fearful, or resentful about epilepsy. Or are crises or disappointments in your life that are not related to epilepsy draining energy away from controlling your epilepsy and preventing you from making positive changes in your life? For example, sometimes marital problems or poverty can overwhelm a person and lead him to give up on everything in life.

Lack of motivation is of concern when it alters important life functions, such as caring for oneself or dependents, relating with family and friends, or performing at school or work. If the problem continues for a long period—six months to a year—it is crucial that you realize action is needed.

HOW DO I KNOW IF I MIGHT BENEFIT FROM PROFESSIONAL COUNSELING?

Many people resist any suggestion that they might benefit from talking with a professional counselor, such as a psychologist or psychiatrist. This is understandable, because in our society the one thing we are expected to be most in control of is our minds. As we grow more knowledgeable about the complexity of the mind and human behavior, however, this attitude is changing. Our society is beginning to realize the tremendous benefits that can come from talking with a professional who has been educated to identify underlying problems and to help people find solutions.

The odds are that you don't need professional counseling. But that does not mean you can't benefit from an initial discussion that will help you decide whether to continue working with a professional counselor. At that initial meeting, you and your counselor will probably focus on issues such as:

- How concerned are you about your problem(s)?
- What impact are these problem(s) having on your life?
- Is anyone close to you concerned about these problems and/or the effects they are having on your life?

After discussing these issues, the question of whether or not to seek professional help is totally up to you. Keep in mind that it is common for people with life challenges such as epilepsy to benefit from occasional counseling. The rate of major depression, for example, is about twice as high in people with epilepsy as it is in the general population. So if you decide to pursue counseling, you are not alone. Congratulate yourself for taking that important first step in improving your life.

WHAT ARE SOME COMMON PROBLEMS FACING PEOPLE WITH EPILEPSY?

One of the most common subjects of concern for anyone, including people with epilepsy, is a problem establishing relationships with others. Because of the complexity of human behavior and the communication age in which we live, this is a universal concern. However, it does not become any less complex when just two individuals are involved, as anyone knows who has just tried to make a new friend.

If you have problems meeting people, ask yourself what is keeping you from becoming more social. Is it that you might have to tell the person you have epilepsy, or that you might have a seizure in front of him? If so, realize that these fears are standing in the way of your meeting and becoming close to other people. A counselor might be able to help you learn about and overcome these fears.

If you are able to discuss your epilepsy with other people, yet you still cannot seem to establish friendships or close relationships, it may help to consider how you present yourself. When you meet someone new, is epilepsy one of the first things that comes up? If so, it may be better for you to focus on something you have in common. Give the other person a chance to learn about you and your interests. Then, when the time seems right, discuss the fact that you have epilepsy, and explain how you control it and cope with its challenges. In this light, most people will tend to admire a person who confronts a major life challenge.

Some people with epilepsy choose not to discuss the disorder with a new acquaintance, especially in relationships with the opposite sex. Then, when they begin dating, they may never get around to revealing that they have epilepsy. This is a personal judgment that each person with epilepsy has to make. However, it can be very damaging to a personal relationship if a seizure occurs without the other person being prepared for it. It may be much less traumatic if the possibility of a seizure has been discussed and the other person is prepared to deal with it and accept it.

Perhaps the most important, yet hardest, thing to avoid when meeting another person is making assumptions. In other words, if things don't work out between you, don't assume that your epilepsy is to blame. There are many reasons two people might not get along. If you are pleasant and share your interests with the other person, you have done all anyone can do to establish a friendship. If, upon learning later that you have epilepsy, the other person ends the relationship, that tells you something about the person's character. On the other hand, epilepsy will likely be a factor in a friendship or romantic relationship. It is usually far less important than things such as mutual interests and physical attraction. However, the other person may be fearful of not knowing what to do if you have a seizure, or may have grown up with negative images about epilepsy. If you are comfortable discussing your epilepsy, you can be open and counter any fears or apprehensions. If he still does not want to associate with you, that tells you one of two things: either he doesn't want to be friends with you for other reasons, or he feels strongly enough about your epilepsy to rule out any relationship with you. In either case, it is best to accept this decision and attempt to meet someone else.

Some people with epilepsy have lived or are living in isolated home or supervised living situations. They may not have had much contact with other people, especially those who do not have epilepsy. In this case, it may be helpful to establish social relationships in a group situation, such as a support group, a recreational club, a religious group, or a political or social advocacy organization. By meeting several people and sharing interests and activities with them, it may be easier to, when appropriate, discuss epilepsy and establish personal relationships.

HOW CAN I BECOME MORE INDEPENDENT FROM MY PARENTS OR GROUP HOME?

Wanting to be independent is the essence of becoming an adult. Like every adult situation, independence involves many complex rights as well as responsibilities. It can be a scary but enriching experience—both at the same time. Each person's situation is a little different, depending on what type of lifestyle he has had as a child and adolescent, and on how well his epilepsy is controlled.

Like achieving any goal, becoming independent involves many small steps. Discuss with your parents or guardian a plan to achieve a goal, such as getting your own apartment. Don't let yourself be upset by objections they may have at first. Letting go is hard for all parents, and it is even harder for parents of a son or daughter with a disorder such as epilepsy. They may fear that you will not be able to manage your epilepsy without them, or that you will not be able to make it on your own. It is important to discuss each of their specific fears, with each person listening to and accepting the worth of the other person's point of view. Then try to work together on a plan that includes specific small steps and a timetable for them. The more support each person can give the other, the more likely it is that this plan will succeed to everyone's satisfaction.

If a parent or guardian is not willing to discuss your desire for independence, it may help to include a third party in the discussion. This could be your doctor, nurse, counselor, social worker, a close relative, or a member of the clergy. This outside observer can look at your situation from an objective point of view, with less emotion than those directly involved. Working together, it may be possible to reach an agreeable solution.

Sometimes, even though your parents agree that it's important for you to live more independently, there may still be barriers. For example, it is often difficult to be able to afford to pay for rent, especially if you are unemployed. Some individuals with epilepsy may not be able to live alone, but it can be difficult to find a roommate or the proper type of assistance. In these situations, it can be helpful to obtain the opinion of a social worker or other professional who might be able to provide you with information regarding financial assistance and the types of living arrangements available in your community.

Most importantly, don't give up on something you feel strongly about. You will need to prove that you can handle each step. The best way to succeed is to focus on one step at a time rather than letting yourself get frustrated by delays in reaching your overall goal.

IS THERE ANY LINK BETWEEN EPILEPSY AND VIOLENT BEHAVIOR?

There is no scientific or medical evidence that epilepsy causes violent behavior. Some books and films, and even some murder trials, have attempted to link violence and epilepsy. No direct link has ever been proved. Of course, people with epilepsy sometimes become violent, just as people without epilepsy sometimes do.

There are several reasons why some people link epilepsy and violent behavior. First, both epilepsy and violence involve temporary episodes of loss of self-control. Second, sometimes a person having a seizure will swear or make a fist, or react violently if restrained. However, there is no evidence that these acts are directed against anyone. There is no need to fear being attacked by a person just because he has seizures.

EEG measurements of people who commit violent acts have failed to reveal any link between violent behavior and EEG changes such as those that occur during a seizure. This does not mean that a person with epilepsy will never act violently, however. Violent behavior may be caused by many things in life. Anyone who loses self-control and becomes violent should be evaluated and helped to prevent further such acts.

HOW CAN I GET OVER FEELING ANGRY AND DEPRESSED?

Everyone feels angry and depressed at times. Usually there is a good reason for these feelings, and they go away when the reason is no longer there. Whether or not the feelings persist, it helps to talk about them with another person. Negative feelings are very real to the person experiencing them. Talking about them with another person, such as a family member, friend, spouse, clergyperson, or psychologist can help the person see that he is focusing too much on negative things, or that the feelings are unrealistic.

There is no reason to be overly concerned about feeling angry or depressed unless you cannot get over the feeling yourself or by talking with someone close to you. Most people expect or hope that problems will solve themselves, and this sometimes does happen. But sometimes it can help to try to step back from the problem and think about it and how it could be solved. For example, it might help to make a list of things that bother you, and then to write down steps you could take to solve these problems. Make a plan for taking those steps and evaluating the results. Anger can be caused by something a person can't change, such as epilepsy. It can still help to acknowledge that you are angry about it, and then to focus on things you can change.

Talking with someone whose judgment and advice you respect can also be helpful. Try to be as open as possible, both when telling the other person your feelings and concerns, and when listening to that person's feelings and suggestions. Take advantage of any help or support he or someone else can give you, and return that support. Accepting and giving support is the foundation of a strong relationship.

Negative feelings can interfere with your life, preventing you from holding a job, causing problems in your marriage or family, affecting friendships, or interfering with efforts to achieve goals. If any of these happens, you might discuss it with your doctor. Either the doctor can help you or suggest that you meet with a professional counselor. In an initial meeting with a counselor you will be able to discuss some of the problems you are having, as well as how you might benefit from further meetings. A counselor can be especially helpful if there is no one you feel you can discuss your problems and share your feelings with.

Feelings can be affected by many things that aren't always obvious. Two major factors are a person's self-esteem and self-concept, which are closely related to whether someone most often feels happy, optimistic, angry, or depressed. Self-concept is your feeling of who you are and how you are unique as a person, while self-esteem is the inner sense of personal value and worth that you have developed throughout your life.

How you feel about yourself can change as your life changes. When your epilepsy is under control, you may take pride in the different parts of your life and your roles, such as being a father or mother, a musician, or an artist. But if you start to have seizures more frequently, your self-concept may change so that you mainly think of yourself as a person with epilepsy. This can cause anger or depression and low self-esteem. If your self-concept and self-esteem remain negative, these feelings may cause major problems.

For example, perhaps you are feeling anxious or fearful about meeting others socially. This may lead you to avoid doing things that would require some contact with other people, such as going to dances or joining a club, even if you really would like to do them. You might become depressed about this or angry when anyone mentions your lack of participation. This may also cause you to avoid making long-term commitments to others, even though you would like to share plans with them. It is these types of underlying problems that can consistently set off chain reactions of feelings and interfere with your lifestyle.

Sometimes it is very hard to understand why problems are occurring in your life. If you choose to seek professional help, you and your counselor may try to find ways to improve your self-esteem and self-concept. The counselor may suggest that a spouse, other family member, or close friend become involved in the discussions. This is not an attempt to get criticism of your actions or feelings. It is an attempt to consider all factors and views about your life. The counselor can keep discussions on a positive note and can sometimes help people recognize or plan solutions to their problems. By trying specific new behaviors or ways of looking at things, you may be able to overcome problems with anxiety, anger, or depression.

If depression persists and overwhelms you, it is extremely important that you seek professional help. Major depression is twice as common in people with epilepsy as in the general public and the rate of suicide is higher. This tragedy can be prevented by watching for warning signs, such as change in appetite, sleep disruption, pulling back from social encounters, feeling very pessimistic or fearful, no longer enjoying things that usually give pleasure, and thinking or talking about suicide. A psychologist or psychiatrist can be helpful in treating depression and reducing the risk of suicide.

HOW CAN FAMILY MEMBERS HELP A PERSON OVERCOME SOCIAL AND PSYCHOLOGICAL PROBLEMS?

Family members can be a person's greatest support group. Unfortunately, they can also be a negative influence. Family relationships are usually complex. If the family takes a positive approach to helping a member become independent and live well, the result will usually be positive. But if the family is too critical or pessimistic about a member's abilities, the person with epilepsy may face major problems. And if parents and siblings are overprotective and do things that the person with epilepsy could do by himself, he may remain dependent and live a less full and productive life.

If you are not happy with the way things are going in your family, take the time to discuss, in a positive way, things that could be changed. Ask how others are feeling about the family, and find out if there are ways each member could help others. Sometimes little things are the underlying causes of serious conflicts. By finding out what they are, a family can deal with them and either prevent or begin to solve bigger problems. If other family members are not willing to discuss things, let them know that you will be there if and when they are willing to talk. This may give them some time to think about the situation, and they may either take steps to make it better or finally decide to discuss it with you.

Sometimes family problems have been developing for so long that it is hard for members to see problems or understand why they are occurring. Often families can benefit from professional counseling just as much as individuals can. Epilepsy adds a series of complex problems to the stressors that families usually experience. By taking a positive approach to overcoming these stressors, families can live well, and in so doing, they can help a person with epilepsy live well.

The next two chapters will discuss other concerns for adults—sexuality and pregnancy.

15

Sexuality and the Person with Epilepsy

Ilo E. Leppik, M.D., and Doug G. Heck, Ph.D.

Sexuality is a natural part of everyone's life. Each of us must learn how to express the sexual part of himself, just as we all must learn how to deal with the responsibilities involved. And, at various times in our lives, each of us will make decisions and have concerns about dating, sexual expression, marriage, and having children.

In general, epilepsy has little or no effect on an individual's sexual and reproductive abilities. However, people with epilepsy may have some special concerns and obligations as they experience each of these life events. This chapter answers questions that people with epilepsy commonly ask about sexuality. We hope this general information will prompt individuals to ask specific questions of their doctors. If you are concerned about your situation, your doctor can help you or direct you to the appropriate professional for help and advice.

WHAT EFFECT DOES EPILEPSY HAVE ON SEXUAL FUNCTION?

Epilepsy and its treatment ordinarily do not have any effect on sexual or reproductive functions. And, likewise, there is no evidence that sexual activity of any kind has any effect on epilepsy or the frequency of seizures. In rare cases, sexual excitement seems sometimes to cause a seizure. Many emotional factors related to sexual activity could be contributing to seizures in such cases. Discuss this with your doctor if it seems to be a problem for you.

While most people with epilepsy are perfectly normal sexually, sexual desire may be reduced if the person with epilepsy is oversedated (drowsy or very relaxed) from taking an antiepileptic medication or other medicine. Occasionally, this is the first sign of oversedation. If you are bothered or worried by a reduced desire for sex, inform your doctor. Counseling may help you take steps to change it. If the problem is caused by your medication, it may be possible to reduce the dosage or switch to another.

It is important to realize that not everyone has the same sexual needs or desires. Don't judge yourself by the examples portrayed on television and in movies. There is no good or bad when it comes to amount of sexual activity. Each of us must evaluate what feels right for our own situation. Putting too much pressure on oneself—or yielding to pressure from someone else—only makes a problem out of what is probably a normal situation. It also makes it harder to meet other people and establish healthy relationships.

If you are not currently dating, or if you are just beginning to date, it is natural to have many concerns and anxieties. Epilepsy can add an extra hurdle to what can be a trying but very rewarding pursuit of a friend and lover. More than half the people with epilepsy develop the disorder before they reach adulthood. This means that a great many teenagers and young adults with epilepsy have faced the challenge of dating. This was discussed in Chapter 13, but it is obviously very pertinent to the subject of sexuality.

Few of us find it easy to meet new people and form lasting relationships. Putting too much emphasis on the sexual part of a budding friendship can ruin what could have been a lifelong relationship. Don't make the mistake of losing what is good about yourself by trying to mimic the "sexy" behavior portrayed in the media. If you feel good about who you are, and if you continue to try to meet people with interests similar to your own, you will succeed.

Probably everyone's biggest fear about dating is being rejected. Since many people with epilepsy already feel rejected by society, this is a particular issue for them. Whether it is being refused when asking someone for a date, not being noticed by someone you are hoping will show interest in you, or having a relationship end when you would like it to develop further, everyone experiences the hurt of rejection at some time in life. This is the risk anyone takes when pursuing the tremendous benefits of emotional attachment to another person. Some people interpret one or a few experiences with rejection as proof that they are not capable of being liked or loved.

Likewise, people with epilepsy may think that because of their disorder, they will never be able to have a loving relationship or experience sexuality. It is a mistake to let these feelings prevent any further attempts at dating or intimacy. It may help to discuss this problem with parents or a counselor, who may help analyze the experience so that you can learn from it. It is never easy to go on and face the risk of further rejection, but it is the only way to develop one's ability to establish close relationships with another person.

If you have not had any luck dating, or if you have few chances to meet other people, it is probably best to begin with group activities. This will help you get to know individuals better, and it may be possible to get a better sense of whether someone likes you enough to go on a date. Then, by gradually sharing things about yourself, including your epilepsy, you can grow closer to the other person, and possibly develop an intimate relationship. Don't put too much emphasis on sexuality right away or pressure the other person into physical contact. Let yourself and the other person become comfortable with each other, and then if trust, affection, and love develop it will be easier to discuss the sexual aspect of your relationship.

When to begin sexual relations is a matter for each individual to decide. Everyone has to learn about sexual activity, birth control, and sexually transmitted diseases. There are many good books available at your book store to help you learn. If one engages in sexual activity without desiring children, then one is responsible for preventing unwanted pregnancy. With current birth control methods, there is little excuse for such an occurrence. Discuss with your doctor the most effective and appropriate form of birth control for you.

For several reasons, a person with epilepsy must be especially aware of the possibility of pregnancy. First, antiepileptic medications—just like many other medications—may cause birth defects. The fetus is most likely to be harmed in the first two months of pregnancy, when its organs are developing. This is before most women know they are pregnant. That is why it is so important for a woman with epilepsy to have a planned pregnancy. She, her husband, and doctor must work together to maximize the safety of epilepsy treatment, both for herself and for the baby. Risk can be reduced with planning and careful obstetrical and neurological management. See the next chapter for information about planning and having a successful pregnancy.

Another reason to avoid an unwanted pregnancy is the extra responsibilities involved in raising a child. Supporting and caring for a baby place many strains on a person and on a couple. These responsibilities may be overwhelming if they are added to other stressful factors, such as financial problems or poorly controlled epilepsy. We all owe it to our children, and to ourselves, to consider seriously our ability to raise a healthy, wanted, and loved child.

IS IT POSSIBLE FOR A WOMAN WITH EPILEPSY TO HAVE HEALTHY CHILDREN?

More than 90% of women with epilepsy have normal, healthy babies. It is important, however, to discuss this with a doctor who has experience with epilepsy and pregnancy. This planning must take place before a couple has unprotected intercourse, and especially before the woman finds out she is pregnant. The next chapter will explain why this is so important.

16

Planning for a Successful Pregnancy

Mark S. Yerby, M.D., M.P.H., and Ilo E. Leppik, M.D.

Planning a pregnancy is important for every woman, but it is especially crucial for women with epilepsy. As we explained in the previous chapter, irreversible damage can be done to a fetus before a woman even knows she is pregnant. The woman, her husband, and her doctor must work together before a pregnancy to maximize the safety of the epilepsy treatment, both for the woman and the baby.

This chapter will discuss the steps involved in planning for pregnancy, as well as some of the concerns women with epilepsy and their husbands have about pregnancy.

HOW SOON SHOULD PREGNANCY PLANNING START?

Planning should start before a woman becomes sexually active. If the woman decides to have intercourse, but does not want to become pregnant, her doctor, nurse, or a Planned Parenthood or other clinic can help her and her partner choose a suitable form of contraception.

When a married couple decide they want to have a baby—but before they stop using contraception—they should first arrange a meeting with the doctor managing her epilepsy. That doctor might want to make changes in her treatment program, or might refer her to a neurologist who has experience managing epilepsy during pregnancy and/or to an obstetrician who has experience managing pregnancy in women with epilepsy. It might take several months to adjust medication, evaluate seizure control, and maximize her health before the couple can safely stop using contraception. Then, as soon as she notices signs of pregnancy, she should make an appointment with the doctor or doctors who will be helping her have a successful pregnancy.

IF I BECOME PREGNANT, SHOULD I DISCONTINUE MY ANTIEPILEPTIC MEDICATIONS?

No. If you are already pregnant, it is more dangerous for you and for your baby if you stop taking your medications. Women with epilepsy usually need to be treated with antiepileptic medication during pregnancy, unless they have been seizure-free for a number of years. Ideally, it is best not to take any medication while you are pregnant, but in reality, most women with epilepsy will have seizures when they discontinue their medications. Status epilepticus can occur with a sudden stop of medications, and in a recent survey of 29 reported cases of status epilepticus in pregnant women, there were nine deaths among the mothers and 14 fetal deaths.

The time to ask your doctor if it may be possible to reduce or discontinue your medication is before you attempt to have a baby. That way you and your doctor will have time to evaluate how safe and effective this will be. For a woman with epilepsy, pregnancy is best planned with a neurologist who is familiar with this special situation. Whether you can safely discontinue your antiepileptic medications during pregnancy is a decision that is best made by your neurologist. If it is not safe, he can adjust the medication to the most effective dosage. The doctor can also help you become as healthy as possible in other areas of your life, such as nutrition and stress management.

As your pregnancy progresses, the level of antiepileptic medication in your blood may gradually decline, even though you are taking the same dose. For this reason, your doctor may need to increase your dosage to protect you from having seizures.

IS TAKING TWO OR THREE DIFFERENT ANTIEPILEPTIC MEDICATIONS MORE DANGEROUS DURING PREGNANCY THAN TAKING JUST ONE?

Taking more than one antiepileptic medication has been associated with an increased rate of major and minor birth defects. This does not prove that these medications cause the birth defects. It is possible that the women who require multiple drugs to control their seizures may have a more severe form of epilepsy that is more likely to be associated with birth defects.

The preferred treatment for each individual with epilepsy is to take the least number of different medications that is effective at controlling the seizures. This is especially true for women who want to become pregnant. Your neurologist will need to determine if it is safe to reduce the number of medications you take.

WHAT IS THE RISK OF BIRTH DEFECTS IN BABIES OF WOMEN WITH EPILEPSY?

All women have a 2–3% risk of having a child with a birth defect. Children born to women with epilepsy have about a 4–6% risk of being born with a malformation, or about twice the risk when compared to children in the general population. Even so, there is still at least a 90% chance that a woman with epilepsy will have a perfectly normal and healthy child. The cause for the increased risk of birth defects has not been determined. Possible causes include genetic errors related to whatever is causing the woman's epilepsy, effects of antiepileptic medications, or genetic susceptibility to possible harmful effects of the medications.

Whatever the reason for the increased risk of birth defects, the incidence is not high enough to support general recommendations that women with epilepsy should avoid pregnancy, or that they should terminate a pregnancy if it occurs. However, if a 4–6% risk of having a child with a malformation is unacceptable to you, it is important for you to make a decision with which you will feel comfortable.

The most common major malformations noted in the children of women with epilepsy are cleft lip/palate and cardiac defects. Abnormalities of the skeletal, genitourinary, gastrointestinal, and central nervous systems may also occur.

Minor malformations may include a combination of unusual facial features, such as wide-set eyes, flat nasal bridge, small upturned nose, and tiny fingernails and toenails. The facial features usually have no medical significance, and the fingernails and toenails tend to grow normally as the child grows older.

A small head circumference and delayed development have also been reported to occur at a higher rate in the babies of women with epilepsy. The smaller average head circumference usually has no medical significance. In one study, the babies of mothers who took only one antiepileptic medication did not show any developmental delay. The babies of mothers who had to take more than one kind of antiepileptic medication did show some developmental delay, but most caught up to their peers by the age of three.

It may be that by exposing babies to many different stimuli, such as bright colors, activity, speech, and holding, you may be able to reduce any of the effects antiepileptic medications may have on development. This has not been proven, but the extra attention certainly can't hurt your baby.

As we discuss these possible problems, you may again wonder if it is safe to take your medications. You must remember that these problems occur in a small number of babies of mothers who have epilepsy. Further, it is not certain that antiepileptic medications caused them. With your doctor's help, you need to weigh the risks of taking your medication against the risk of not taking it. If you do not take your medication, you will probably have seizures, which may be harmful to you and your unborn child.

IS THERE ANYTHING I CAN DO TO REDUCE ANY RISKS TO MY BABY?

The most important thing you can do for yourself and your baby is to see a neurologist and an obstetrician for help in planning your pregnancy. Do this several months before you would like to start trying to become pregnant. Involve your husband or other family members in this planning, because you will need their help in making sure you get enough rest and nutrition during and after your pregnancy. After you are as healthy as possible and your antiepileptic medication is adjusted to your and the neurologist's satisfaction, you are on the right track for a healthy pregnancy.

After you become pregnant, see both your obstetrician and your neurologist at regular intervals—monthly at first and every week in the later months, or more often if symptoms or problems develop. It is important to eat healthy foods so that you gain enough weight but not too much. It is a good idea to begin taking prenatal vitamins even before you become pregnant, in case your body is lacking any vital nutrients. Remember that much of your baby's development will occur in the first six weeks, so you want to be as healthy as possible before that. Make sure your vitamins contain folic acid, because antiepileptic medications can reduce folic acid levels. Low folic acid levels have been associated with birth defects.

Smoking during pregnancy is very bad for babies and can have serious consequences for their health and development. It is also best to avoid alcohol and caffeine, as well as all street drugs, over-the-counter remedies, and any medications not prescribed by the doctor who is supervising your pregnancy.

Try to reduce the stress in your life as much as possible during your pregnancy. Get plenty of rest and sleep, and engage in moderate exercise, such as walking. If your stress level remains high, you might want to learn some relaxation techniques; your physician or nurse can help you with these. And remember to take your medication as prescribed by your doctor. If you have seizures, report them so steps can be taken to prevent or reduce their occurrence.

WILL I HAVE MORE SEIZURES WHEN I AM PREGNANT?

About one-third of women experience an increase in seizure frequency during pregnancy. Factors that contribute to this increase include poor seizure control prior to pregnancy, failure to take antiepileptic medication as prescribed, and lack of sleep. Most women will have the same number of seizures they had before they became pregnant. And a small number of women have fewer seizures during pregnancy, probably because they are practicing more healthy behaviors during this time.

The risk for increased seizures can be reduced if you take certain actions. It is important that you and your physician work together to get your seizures under control before you become pregnant. You need to take your medication regularly—before, during, and after your pregnancy. Getting adequate sleep can be difficult when you are pregnant, especially if you have small children at home. But adequate sleep is very important for your health during pregnancy, and not getting enough sleep can be dangerous if this has caused you to have seizures in the past. It is advantageous to have family and friends to turn to for help during this time.

If you have not done so already, work with your doctor to analyze what has caused you to have seizures in the past. Possible factors might include emotional stress, fatigue, or alcoholic beverages. You will want to make a special effort to avoid these factors once you become pregnant. Keeping a diary, or calendar, of the number and severity of seizures you have each day, along with a record of your medication, will be helpful to you and your physician. It will provide accurate information that will help you and your doctor make decisions about managing your epilepsy. Also, keeping a record of your medication may help you remember to take it, and it will help your doctor evaluate the medication levels in your blood.

IF I HAVE SEIZURES WHEN I AM PREGNANT, WILL THEY HARM MY BABY?

Possibly, but not necessarily. A seizure is not good for the woman or her baby. Although rare, miscarriages have occurred following a single generalized tonic–clonic seizure. This type of seizure can also decrease the fetal heart rate, which can be a sign that the baby is in distress. The reason for the drop in heart rate is not clearly understood. It might be due to decreased oxygen because the mother is not breathing adequately during the seizure, or it may be caused by reduced blood supply to the baby during the seizure, or both.

Generalized tonic–clonic seizures occurring during pregnancy have not been linked to birth defects. But one study did report an increased risk for any adverse outcome if the mother had a seizure during pregnancy. For these reasons, it is important to minimize the number of seizures you have during pregnancy. It is important to take your medications as prescribed and to avoid those things that may cause you to have a seizure, such as lack of sleep or extreme stress.

You should notify your neurologist if you do have a seizure. This does not mean that you should panic or assume that your baby has been harmed. Most babies whose mothers had seizures during pregnancy are perfectly normal. However, it is best to take precautions to minimize any risks to your unborn child.

WILL I HAVE ANY OTHER COMPLICATIONS DURING PREGNANCY OR DELIVERY BECAUSE OF MY EPILEPSY?

The only other pregnancy complication clearly related to epilepsy is an increased risk of vaginal bleeding during and after pregnancy. Early and consistent prenatal care by your obstetrician will improve the chances that any problem will be detected and treated promptly. By avoiding smoking, caffeine, alcohol, drugs, and toxic chemicals such as pesticides, oven cleaners, and paint, you can help to minimize any other complications that might occur.

Women with epilepsy are about twice as likely to have a cesarean section (surgical) delivery rather than a vaginal delivery. The reasons for this are not clear. It is uncommon for a seizure to occur during labor or delivery. Your obstetrician or a nurse will discuss your delivery with you as it progresses. If any special actions are indicated, they will be discussed with you and/or your husband if possible and the doctor will intervene in whatever way he decides is best for you and your baby.

WILL THE MEDICATION I AM TAKING AFFECT MY BABY WHEN IT IS BORN?

When the mother has been taking medications such as phenobarbital, her newborn may act sedated. This can last for a few hours or up to a week. After that time, some babies develop withdrawal symptoms. These may consist of irritability, tremors, vomiting, poor sucking, fast breathing, and sleep disturbances. One or more of these symptoms may last from a few days to about three months. These problems can be frustrating to parents, but they do improve and are seldom serious unless they interfere with the baby's ability to get enough to eat. If your baby fails to gain weight properly, an evaluation by a pediatrician may be needed.

There is also a small risk that a baby of a mother who takes antiepileptic medication may develop a bleeding disorder within the first 24 hours after birth. Experts recommend that the mother take vitamin K1 during the last two weeks of pregnancy to help prevent this from occurring. Your obstetrician can prescribe this for you.

WILL I BE ABLE TO BREASTFEED MY BABY IF I AM TAKING ANTIEPILEPTIC MEDICATIONS?

Yes. Only small amounts of some antiepileptic medications are excreted into the breast milk, compared to large amounts of others. The average percentages of drug level in the breast milk for some common antiepileptic medications are: Depakote, 10%; Tegretol, 40–60%; Dilantin, 60%; phenobarbital, 80%; and Mysoline, 60%. You may still breastfeed if you are taking *one* of the medications with a higher concentration in the breast milk.

You should be particularly cautious if you take phenobarbital and Mysoline together, or if you take ethosuximide (Zarontin), since high levels of these drugs have been measured in the breast milk. Although most babies suffer no ill effects, if your baby fails to eat or gain weight as expected, check with your pediatrician.

WHAT IF I HAVE A SEIZURE WHILE I'M HOLDING MY BABY?

This is a possibility, so plan for what you will do in case you have a seizure while attending to the baby. If you have a warning when you are about to have a seizure, you can plan a safe area in each room, where you can safely lay the baby down when you feel a seizure coming on.

Some persons do not have a warning before seizures, but others learn to recognize a sign or may not feel right for several hours before they have a seizure. If you have this kind of warning, you may wish to have a friend or family member stay with you for that day.

Taking your medication as prescribed is the most important factor in reducing your chances of having a seizure. During the weeks after delivery your neurologist will want to check your antiepileptic drug levels to make sure they are in the desired range. Even though you are taking the same amount of medication as you were before delivery, your blood levels may rise in the weeks following delivery. Your neurologist or nurse will be able to tell you what symptoms might indicate that your blood levels of medication are too high.

In addition to taking your medication, there are other ways to reduce the risk of seizures. It is important to get adequate sleep at night and not get too physically tired during the day. All new mothers appreciate the help of family members or friends when adjusting to a new baby. You may need to learn to sleep when the baby sleeps, which may be difficult if you have other small children and no one to help you.

Family members may be able to help you during the night by taking turns with feedings. If you breastfeed, you may be able to pump some of your breast milk into bottles during the day and place it in the refrigerator for warming and feeding by someone else during the night.

In at least one study, seizures were more likely to occur in the weeks after a baby is born. This can be a stressful time. Your body has been stressed by the processes of labor and delivery. You may be excited or anxious. Your hormones are changing. You may have difficulty getting enough rest or sleep. Share these feelings with your doctor or nurse. They may be able to suggest solutions. Or they may know of other women with epilepsy who have children, and you could talk with them about how they handled various practical situations.

WHAT ARE THE CHANCES THAT MY BABY WILL HAVE EPILEPSY?

Babies of mothers who have epilepsy have about a 3% chance of developing epilepsy. If the father has epilepsy and the mother does not, the chance that the baby will develop epilepsy is less. This is about the same chance that any individual in the population has of developing epilepsy. If both the mother and the father have epilepsy, the baby's chance of developing the disorder is slightly higher than 3%.

A CHECKLIST FOR A HEALTHY BABY

If you have epilepsy and must take antiepileptic medication, your chances of having a normal baby are high—at least 90% and more commonly around 94%. You can help your baby by adhering to the following guidelines for providing the best possible environment for your baby to develop.

1. Plan your pregnancy. See your neurologist and obstetrician/gynecologist *before* you become pregnant.
2. Make an appointment with your obstetrician when you first suspect you are pregnant. Keep regular appointments with your obstetrician and neurologist throughout your pregnancy.
3. Take your antiepileptic medication as prescribed by your doctor.
4. Reduce, as best you can, any factors in your life that usually make a seizure more likely to occur.
5. Report any seizures promptly to your neurologist.
6. Get plenty of rest and sleep.
7. Eat enough healthy foods so that you gain weight during your pregnancy. If you have financial problems that make this difficult, ask a social worker about federally funded programs, such as WIC, for mothers and infants.

8. Take prenatal vitamins with folic acid before and during your pregnancy. Ask your doctor to prescribe vitamin K1 during the last few weeks of your pregnancy.
9. DO NOT SMOKE. Smoking is harmful to the baby during all months of pregnancy.
10. Avoid beverages with caffeine or alcohol.
11. Do not take any street drugs such as marijuana, cocaine, and speed, and avoid toxic chemicals such as paint, oven cleaner, and pesticides.
12. Do not take any medication, including medications you can buy at the drugstore without a prescription, unless approved by your doctor.

17

Epilepsy in the Workplace

Judy L. Antonello, M.S.W., A.C.S.W., and Doug G. Heck, Ph.D.

Having a job is a powerful contributor to self-esteem. Besides helping a person gain financial independence, working opens up many social and recreational avenues. While some people with frequent seizures may not be able to hold a job, most people with epilepsy can work with few—if any—restrictions. Almost every field of employment is open to people with epilepsy, so it is a mistake to let the disorder dash any hopes for a career. With proper education and job training, people with epilepsy can be as successful or more so than anyone else in the workplace.

This chapter discusses questions we are sometimes asked about career planning, training programs, and what to tell employers and fellow employees about epilepsy.

WHAT LIMITS DOES EPILEPSY PLACE ON CAREER PLANNING?

Very few occupations have restrictions that make them unavailable to people with epilepsy, and some of those restrictions that currently exist are being modified as antiepileptic medications improve control of seizures. It is always a good idea to check out whether any existing restrictions might apply to you.

For example, people with epilepsy are not eligible for military service, unless they have been off medications and seizure-free for at least five years. However, the military will accept people in some noncombat, specialized areas, such as medicine and dentistry. Young men with epilepsy must register for selective service.

Occupations in public transportation (pilot, train engineer, bus driver) and interstate trucking are closed to people with epilepsy, because they involve sole responsibility for others' safety.

Safety concerns may limit the options for a person with epilepsy in some other areas, such as working with dangerous machinery, being a police officer or fire fighter, or driving a vehicle. Any limitations in these areas depend on how well a person's seizures are controlled and how well qualified he is for the job.

Everyone can benefit from career planning, starting in high school and possibly continuing throughout life as one's desires or situation changes. For a high school student, career planning is mostly a matter of seeking information on various occupations of interest, while keeping open as many options as possible. This is not the time for a student to rule out careers or professions because he is having frequent seizures. Seizure control may improve with more intensive seizure management or with the development of new medical options for people with epilepsy. More directed planning can take place once it is apparent that seizure control has been stabilized.

All high school students deserve the benefit of social and educational counseling that will help them make the most of their intellectual abilities, talents, and skills. As a student nears graduation, decisions will need to be made about going to college or vocational school, or about getting a job. Epilepsy will have some bearing on these decisions, but it is important that options not be ruled out without input from the student's doctor and professionals familiar with career planning for people with epilepsy. We will describe these services later in this chapter.

CAN AN EMPLOYER REFUSE TO HIRE ME JUST BECAUSE I HAVE EPILEPSY?

Not in most states, which have enacted laws protecting the employment rights of people with medical handicaps. The federal government has a similar law covering all federal employment and jobs with companies or organizations that receive federal funds or have federal contracts. These laws prohibit refusing to hire or firing a person with a medical handicap without a valid reason (for example, a legitimate safety issue). Of course, you must meet all other requirements for the job, and you needn't be selected over more qualified applicants for a position.

As noted, safety issues may be a legitimate factor in a hiring decision. However, most states require an employer to cite specific and realistic safety concerns in making a decision not to hire or to fire a person with epilepsy. Be honest with yourself in evaluating whether your seizures might pose a safety hazard in the job you are seeking. Be ready to discuss how you would perform the job safely and what you would do in case of a seizure. If you are refused employment because of safety concerns, you must decide if and how to challenge that decision.

Don't be too quick to conclude that you've been turned down because of epilepsy. Remember that most people must apply for many jobs before they are hired. You have a right to ask why you were not hired, and asking can provide valuable information for future job interviews.

If you do suspect that you've been discriminated against, you may want to contact your local affiliate of the Epilepsy Foundation of American (EFA) for advice. They may have a social worker or counselor you can meet with, or they may refer you to another agency. You may then decide to contact your state human rights commission or similar body with a different name. A representative of this group will ask you to file a complaint, and then—possibly after checking with the employer—will tell you if he thinks you have been discriminated against. If so, he will help you to negotiate a solution with the employer and will advise you about legal options if this fails. It may take several months for the human rights commission to investigate your case, so it is a good idea to seek advice from the EFA first.

WHAT SHOULD I SAY ABOUT EPILEPSY WHEN I APPLY FOR A JOB?

It's not a good idea to hide epilepsy when applying for a job. Your employer is likely to find out anyway if health insurance is provided or if you have a seizure at work. You might then be fired for not having provided this information, even if epilepsy would not have prevented your being hired in the first place. Being open about your seizures with your boss and fellow employees can be much easier than worrying that you will have a seizure or that they will find out some other way.

This situation is similar to deciding what to tell new acquaintances about your epilepsy. You don't want people—especially a prospective employer—to judge you based on the fact that you have seizures without knowing anything else about you. Therefore, it is sometimes helpful to omit the fact that you have epilepsy from a job application form. If it asks about medical conditions, indicate that you are willing to discuss this part of the application in an interview.

Before an interview, prepare yourself for questions about your epilepsy. Some states limit the types of questions that can be asked about medical conditions in a job interview. You can get this information from your state department of employment services or from your local affiliate of the EFA. However, you should be prepared to describe briefly what epilepsy is, what type of seizures you have, how often they occur, whether they occur at certain times of day or in certain situations, whether you have any warning (aura), and how long it takes you to recover.

Most interviewers will be sensitive when asking questions about an applicant's health. They will be most concerned about how a particular disorder will affect your ability to do the job safely and well. Be sure to discuss your qualifications fully and confidently. Then tell the interviewer how you cope with the possibility of seizures. It is natural to be nervous, so don't feel that you're any different for that reason. The best way to appear confident about yourself is to make frequent eye contact with the interviewer, and to talk in a cheerful, positive way about the assets you think you can bring to the organization.

A few interviewers may go directly to any information that is missing from an application. Some may even express negative opinions about your ability to handle the job. This type of interviewer is probably reacting on the basis of a bad past experience with an employee's health problem, or on the basis of misinformation about epilepsy. The best way to overcome this type of reaction is to be ready with facts about epilepsy and the different types of seizures. Try not to react defensively to the interviewer, because he may use your reaction as a reason not to hire you. Explain the facts about your seizures and how you would prevent them from interfering with your ability to do the job in question. Add that you expect to be evaluated just like any other employee. Also mention that there are thousands of people with epilepsy who are employed and doing well in all types of jobs and careers.

Some employers may be afraid that their Worker's Compensation insurance rates may increase if they hire a person with epilepsy. This is not true, because the Worker's Compensation premiums of all but the largest companies are based on the overall accident rates in their industry, not on the medical histories of a company's employees. Besides, a Department of Labor study found that workers with epilepsy actually had slightly better safety records, perhaps because they tend to be particularly careful. In addition, some states provide "second injury" funds that limit employer liability for accidents that may occur among workers with disabilities or disorders, including epilepsy. You can get information about "second injury" coverage from your local EFA affiliate or your state Worker's Compensation department.

It is helpful in any job interview to provide references from people who are familiar with you as a person, and with the way you cope with epilepsy. This may include teachers, coaches, clergymen, and especially former employers. Many interviewers will ask if they can contact your doctor. To be prepared for this, first discuss with your doctor how your epilepsy may affect your ability to perform the type of job you are seeking. If he thinks that you would do well, ask him to write a letter, and to respond to calls from any prospective employers. This is probably the most effective way to reassure an employer that your epilepsy will not endanger yourself or others, and that you will be able to meet the demands of the job.

What you tell fellow employees about epilepsy depends largely on what type of work you do, how often you have seizures, and how comfortable you feel sharing this information. It is a good idea to discuss this first with your immediate supervisor, so that you can work out a plan that both of you feel comfortable with. Again, by first giving people a chance to meet you and get to know a little bit about you, you can help them put your epilepsy into proper perspective. Accurate information discussed openly in a relaxed atmosphere is preferable to responding with too little information when it is too late to do any good.

Remember that it is natural for tensions to occur in the workplace over many issues. Epilepsy is just one more variable that may affect how people relate to you. If you sense that a coworker is uncomfortable working with you, find an appropriate time to talk with that person. Get to know him a little better, and then let him know how much you appreciate his willingness to help you. Ask if the person has any questions about epilepsy or about how to respond to a seizure. By being willing to discuss these things, you do two things: First, you show that you are not ashamed of epilepsy and are not trying to get special attention. And, second, you can usually relieve any concerns or misunderstandings the person has about epilepsy. Both of these positive steps go a long way toward making you more successful and comfortable at work.

WHAT FIRST-AID MEASURES ARE NECESSARY IN THE WORKPLACE?

If you work closely with coworkers and there is a chance that you will have a seizure at work, it would be foolish not to provide information that will help them respond correctly to a seizure without overreacting. The most reassuring thing for most people is simply knowing that there is very little they need to do, other than removing objects that may injure you. And you can prevent yourself from being injured by dispelling the myth that it is necessary to force something into the mouth of a person having a seizure.

Discuss your job situation with your supervisor, going over scenarios that might occur if you have a seizure while performing each part of your job. If there are situations that might be dangerous, try to work out satisfactory changes in your duties or in the workplace.

Provide your supervisor and fellow employees with the appropriate sections of Chapter 9, or with seizure first-aid cards available from the Epilepsy Foundation of America, 4351 Garden City Drive, Landover, MD 20785; 301-459-3700 or 800-332-1000. Make sure they understand what type of seizures you might have and are aware of what to do—as well as what not to do. Depending on your job situation, you may decide to speak with coworkers individually or in a group. Whatever you decide is best, be sure to thank them for being understanding and for taking the time to help you be safer on the job.

If you do have a seizure that is witnessed by other employees, discuss it openly with them after you have recovered. Most people find this preferable to acting as if nothing happened, which tends to isolate the person with epilepsy and fuel others' concerns. Since you will probably not be aware of what happened during the seizure, ask witnesses to describe what they saw and how they responded. Ask if they have any questions about the seizure or about first aid. If inappropriate help was given, thank the person but explain specific types of help you would appreciate if you have a seizure in the future. After you have cleared the air of any concern or questions about the seizure, everyone will be much more comfortable getting back into the work routine.

WHAT TYPES OF TRAINING PROGRAMS ARE AVAILABLE FOR PEOPLE WITH EPILEPSY?

The EFA has been very successful in helping people with epilepsy find employment through its Training and Placement Service, or TAPS. Funded by the U.S. Department of Labor, TAPS' mission is to increase and enhance employment of people with epilepsy. TAPS representatives work with applicants and their potential employers to help each feel more comfortable with the other.

TAPS may be able to help you in four ways:

1. Through vocational counseling, TAPS can help you set goals, make choices, and carry out a job search based on your needs and talents.
2. By introducing you to its job clubs, TAPS can bring together job seekers and those who have found jobs to discuss the employment challenges faced by people with epilepsy.
3. TAPS workshops will help you improve your job-seeking skills.
4. By staying in touch with you after you have found a job, TAPS helps you with any problems or concerns you may have.

TAPS also offers employers services such as epilepsy education workshops, phone and personal consultation about specific concerns, and on-the-job training for selected applicants.

Another helpful employment service is the vocational rehabilitation system, which is operated through the federal Rehabilitation Services Administration. Services are offered through each state, so they may differ in the type of help they provide people with epilepsy. In general, the goal is to help people whose disorder or disability limits the type of work they can do, but who can be expected to be able to work after receiving specific vocational training. High school counselors or an EFA representative can refer you to the appropriate state agency in your area.

I'VE BEEN UNEMPLOYED SO LONG I DON'T THINK I'LL EVER BE ABLE TO WORK. WHAT CAN I DO?

Most people prefer to work if at all possible. But, if you have been unemployed for months or years, or if you have never had a job, it can be difficult or frightening to take the steps necessary to find work. If you are afraid that you will lose your disability benefits if you return to work, check with your local Social Security office. Funds are available for disabled people who return to work for a trial period or who have entered a vocational rehabilitation plan. And if you have work expenses related to your epilepsy, they may be deductible from your income. Check with a Social Security counselor about your benefits before accepting a job.

If a vocational counselor has told you that you will probably not be able to hold any kind of job, but you still want to do some kind of work, keep trying. Find out if there is anything you can do to improve your seizure control or to change any other factor that limits your ability to work. In the meantime, you may be able to find some other way to keep busy and help others, such as by doing volunteer work in your community or church. Or you may find partial employment with an agency especially designed to provide work for people who may not be able to hold regular jobs. Ask your vocational counselor about these types of work.

If you have not sought employment counseling or vocational rehabilitation services, ask your doctor or social worker to help you contact the EFA's TAPS program or a state vocational rehabilitation agency. Epilepsy can sometimes prevent a person from working, but in some cases it may become an excuse for not working. Be honest with yourself about your capabilities. A job may open up many social opportunities and greatly increase your self-esteem. If you want to work, there are many people and programs waiting to help you succeed.

18

Obtaining Insurance and Collecting Benefits

Robert J. Gumnit, M.D.

As our society grows increasingly complex, it is becoming more difficult to obtain all the services that can help you live well. Sometimes it may seem more trouble than it is worth to shop for the best insurance and apply for government benefits for yourself and your family. Or, you may feel frustrated and helpless when public employees or private businesses seem to be denying you your legal rights.

This chapter provides suggestions for making the system work for you. This information will be most helpful when put into action by a determined person. This doesn't mean you have to do everything yourself. Much of the battle will be won by finding knowledgeable people to help you. But, to succeed, you will have to be stubbornly insistent on getting the insurance, financial benefits, and rights that are legally yours.

CAN PEOPLE WITH EPILEPSY GET INSURANCE?

Yes, but usually not as easily or cheaply as people who do not have medical disorders or diseases. This may not seem fair, but you have to consider that insurance companies must make a profit. They try to make sure that the premiums paid by policyholders for insurance more than cover all future costs the company will incur, including the administrative costs of running the company.

Insurance companies try to earn a profit by offering insurance at different rates to different groups of people. Their rates are based on the likelihood that a person or family will require payment for covered services, such as medical care, a death benefit, or car repairs. An individual's rates for each type of insurance may depend on factors such as age, current and past health, and driving record. People with epilepsy (and other chronic disorders) are often charged more for health and life insurance than the general population.

Unfortunately, keeping track of group insurance usage by different groups of people is the primary way companies set their rates. However, some will make adjustments for an individual's experience in setting premiums for his policy. This approach is becoming more common as companies realize that epilepsy can often be controlled well.

In general, you have to shop around in order to get the best insurance for the most reasonable cost. When you obtain price quotes from several companies, be sure that each agent is quoting a rate based on the same type and amount of coverage as the others. This can be confusing, so keep asking questions until you understand. It is the insurance company's responsibility to explain exactly what types of coverage you can buy for how much money. Write down this information or obtain a copy from the insurance agent to compare with types of coverage and rates from other companies. If you decide to purchase a policy, the insurance company must provide you with a written explanation of exactly what you have purchased.

Make sure you understand when and how you are supposed to send payments (premiums) for the insurance. And find out exactly how to submit claims for payment. It helps to get to know an individual insurance agent whom you can call with any questions or problems. As the holder of an insurance policy, it is your responsibility to know what your policy covers. You must know how to obtain payment for covered services, and you must file claims according to the procedure set by the company. Sometimes there may be time limits for filing claims, so it is important to obtain and fill out the proper forms promptly. It is also the policyholder's responsibility to pay premiums on a timely basis. Some states require a grace period of 10–14 days for late payments. This means that as long as you send your payment within that time your policy is still in effect. Know the time requirements for your premiums, because if you let your policy lapse you might lose all past and future rights under the insurance.

Before you can shop for insurance, however, you need to know which types are available. The following describe current types of coverage, which may differ depending on where you live, and which will almost certainly change somewhat over the next decade.

Health Insurance

Health insurance is probably the most important type of protection anyone can have, especially people with chronic medical problems. It is also the type that is changing most rapidly in our society, as health costs rise faster than the general rate of inflation. Several types of health insurance are offered by hundreds of companies throughout the United States. The type of insurance may differ drastically from state to state, and between urban and rural areas. (In Chapter 4 we suggested ways to evaluate your current health insurance or to look for new insurance.)

Before you buy a health insurance policy, you will need to know what is covered by each plan and at what cost. If you or a family member has epilepsy, you should pay special attention to whether a policy covers pre-existing conditions, pays for antiepileptic medications and for evaluations by a neurologist, and to any other special needs you may have.

Because there are so many variations in health insurance that change every year in each area of the country, we can't say which type is best for you. The following descriptions consider the relative amount of freedom you will have in obtaining medical care with each type of insurance plan.

Indemnity or Fee-for-Service Health Insurance

This is the traditional kind of health insurance and gives the policyholder the most freedom of choice. If you own this type of insurance, you can choose to see any private doctor at any time, and you can be treated in any hospital you choose. The insurance pays a set percentage (usually 80% of the amount above an annual deductible) of the costs of covered care, and the policyholder pays the rest, called a copayment. Claims must usually be filled out and submitted by the policyholder. If you choose this type of health insurance, be sure that care and medications for epilepsy are covered, and that you can afford to pay the premium. Often the 20% copayment is limited to a certain amount each year so that there is a limit to how much you are responsible for.

Health Maintenance Organizations (HMOs)

HMOs are a type of health "insurance" organization that has grown rapidly in the 1980s. They actually provide a guarantee of services, limited by the contract; this is not the same as insurance, which provides free choice of medical providers and services. There are two main differences between indemnity insurance and HMOs. First, in an HMO you pay a fixed monthly premium that covers all (or nearly all) of your health-care costs without having to submit claims. Second, an HMO restricts you to seeing certain doctors at certain clinics and hospitals.

The theory underlying HMOs is that by organizing hospitals and doctors and paying them set amounts according to how many patients they see and the services they provide, the HMO could keep costs down and provide health care at a reasonable rate. Experts expected HMOs to keep costs as low as possible by encouraging policyholders to use preventative services and by competing with indemnity insurance companies and with each other. It is hard to tell if this has happened, because the costs of new medical technology and an aging population have caused overall health-care costs to rise rapidly even with the competition introduced by HMOs. In most cases HMOs control their costs by avoiding taking on people with pre-existing conditions.

Each type of HMO is organized and operates somewhat differently. These differences can have a drastic impact on a person's ability to obtain high-quality health care, especially for chronic health disorders. They vary widely in how they restrict members' choices of primary doctors, specialists, clinics, and hospitals. The most restrictive type is called a *staff-model HMO*. It will only pay for services provided by doctors at a clinic owned by the HMO, and at a hospital that has a contract with the HMO. In this type of plan, the doctors are employees of the HMO and are usually paid an annual salary plus bonuses according to how many patients they see or how much money the HMO earns that year.

The least restrictive type of HMO is an *IPA model HMO*. This type of HMO is affiliated with independent practitioners. The HMO company signs contracts with private physicians who agree to provide care to HMO members for set fees, plus some type of annual bonus system.

Preferred Provider Organizations

There is a wide range of HMO plans with degrees of member freedom somewhere between the strict staff model and the IPA model. There is also a type of health insurance plan that is a cross between an indemnity plan and an HMO. Called a preferred provider organization (PPO), this type of plan pays all costs of services provided by selected doctors and hospitals. The difference is that a PPO allows members to go to other doctors and hospitals, if they are willing to pay a portion of the costs, usually 20% plus a deductible amount.

Warning: In 1988, an increasing number of HMOs and PPOs declared bankruptcy or were sold to other HMOs, threatening to leave their policy-holders without coverage. In the much longer history of indemnity insurance companies, very few have gone bankrupt. Take these facts into consideration when choosing health insurance.

Medicare

Medicare is a form of health insurance for the elderly (those over age 65) and for younger people who are totally disabled. It is provided and administered by the federal government. There are two parts to Medicare, Part A and Part B. Part A provides coverage of services provided in hospitals, and some nursing home and home-care services for a short time after a patient leaves the hospital. It is financed by employee and employer

Social Security taxes. Part B is voluntary health insurance that partly covers doctor fees, clinic visits, diagnostic tests, and some home health visits. It is financed by a combination of monthly premiums paid by those enrolled and a matching amount from government funds.

The coverage provided by Medicare and the costs to those enrolled change every few years, as the government attempts to stretch the available dollars to meet rising health-care costs. The fact that the average life expectancy is now about 75 years and many more people are living into their 80s and 90s has severely strained Medicare. Medicare cannot be relied on for all health-care needs; for example, it pays very little for long-term care provided in the home or in a nursing home.

Medicaid

Medicaid is comprehensive health insurance for the poor and the near poor. It is funded by a federal subsidy to states, each of which then decides how much state money to contribute and what type of coverage to offer. For this reason, coverage varies greatly in different states, and it can change from year to year based on the financial health of the state.

State Health Insurance Risk Pools

Some states have recognized that people with chronic health disorders are sometimes unable to obtain health insurance or must pay very high rates for coverage. To make insurance available to these people, some states have passed laws requiring all health insurance companies operating in the state to contribute to an organization that provides insurance to those who can't qualify or who must pay a high price for standard health insurance.

For example, in 1976 Minnesota established the Minnesota Comprehensive Health Association (MCHA), which spreads the costs of high-risk insurance among all health insurance agencies in the state. Anyone who has been refused health insurance, whose premiums exceed those available through MCHA, or who has one of the medical conditions covered automatically by MCHA is eligible for coverage. The plan covers 80% of costs over an annual $1,000 deductible per person, and 100% of costs over a $3,000 deductible per person. For those over age 65, a supplement to Medicare is offered.

If you have been refused health insurance or feel that your premiums are too high, check with your state insurance officer, your insurance agent, or your local office of the EFA to find out if your state offers a pooled risk insurance plan.

Life Insurance

Before you shop for life insurance, ask yourself why you want to buy this type of insurance. Not everyone needs life insurance, which provides a benefit for your survivors if you die. And, for those who do buy life insurance, there are vastly different amounts and types that are appropriate. Some people want only to provide enough money for their funerals and burials, whereas others want to leave enough money to protect the financial security of their families. Some people buy life insurance as another type of investment, while for others, the money would be better invested other ways.

The two basic types of life insurance are term life and whole life. The easiest way to describe the difference is that with term life you pay a certain amount to obtain a certain amount of money for your dependents if you die, while whole life is a combination of term life and a savings plan.

Term life insurance is the least expensive. It pays a specific amount in death benefit, and is paid for on an annual rate base. This annual rate may increase as you grow older (annual renewable term), or the rate and amount of insurance may decrease each year (decreasing term). "Term" refers to how many years you agree to pay into the policy—one year, 10 years, or 20 years, for example. At the end of the term you can usually renew the insurance for another term without having to take a physical exam, but be sure to ask your agent about this feature. As with all types of life insurance, term life is cheapest when purchased at a young age. Term life insurance may be provided by an employer, or as a veteran's benefit, or it may be sold along with a home mortgage.

Whole life offers more flexibility than term life insurance, but it also costs more. The amount paid by the policy and the premiums remain the same for the duration of the policy. With inflation, this means that you will be paying much less (in today's dollars) in the final years of the policy. But to receive the death benefit, you may have to keep paying into this type of policy until age 85 or even 100.

The savings account portion of whole life insurance is the most variable of all the options you can choose. In the oldest type, part of your premium pays for your life insurance, and the rest goes into a savings account that earns a low rate of interest. Over the years, this interest rate has not kept up with inflation. You can do two things with this savings account. You can either cancel the policy and withdraw the money in it, or you can borrow against that money at a low interest rate, usually 4–8%. Of course, if you cancel, you would no longer receive a death benefit. And if you die before paying back the money, the unpaid amount will be deducted from your death benefit.

Several new types of whole life insurance have been created in recent years. They are often referred to as *universal life* or *flexible life insurance*.

Basically they offer the policyholder the ability to manage the money in the savings account portion of the policy. Options may include investing in mutual funds, which are investment plans managed by professionals. There is always some amount of risk in these investments, however. If the investments prosper, you may choose to either let your savings account grow accordingly or pay off your policy early. But if the investments lose money or fail to earn a set percentage needed to keep your policy up to date, you may have to pay more into the policy.

Each person should think carefully about whether life insurance is necessary, and if so, what type and how much. Don't let an insurance agent pressure you into buying one type or an amount that you can't afford.

If you are employed and have dependents, it is probably wise to buy some term life insurance (and probably mortgage insurance if you own a home). This will give your family some financial security if you die. You can probably get the most protection for the least money by buying a term policy at a young age and for as long a term as possible. If you are thinking of buying a whole life policy with a savings or investment option, you may want to first consult a financial planner. You may be able to invest your money more safely and more wisely in other ways. Don't rely completely on an insurance agent's advice about financial planning, because they are paid to sell the plans offered by their company.

WHAT TYPES OF SUPPLEMENTAL INCOME BENEFITS ARE AVAILABLE FOR PEOPLE WITH EPILEPSY?

Depending on degree of disability and annual income, people with epilepsy may qualify for benefits under the following plans:

Supplemental Security Income (SSI)

SSI is a federal program run by the Social Security Administration. It pays monthly checks to people who are over 65 or who are totally disabled or blind, and who don't have many personal assets or income. If you are 18 or older, you may qualify for SSI if a physical or mental disability is expected to keep you from working for at least 12 months or is expected to result in death. A child under 18 may get SSI if a disability is as severe as the qualifying adult disability. SSI has strict requirements for covering someone disabled with epilepsy.

Besides disability, SSI requires that a person's resources and income be below a certain level. Resources include real estate, personal belongings, cars, savings and checking accounts, cash, and investments. Some of a parent's resources and income may be counted as belonging to a child who is applying for SSI. The allowable level of resources and income changes annually. To see if you or a family member qualifies for SSI, check with your local Social Security office, which is listed in the telephone directory under "U.S. Government" or "Social Security Administration."

Social Security Disability Income (SSDI)

To qualify for SSDI, you must have worked long enough and recently enough to be insured (dependents can receive benefits under a qualified worker). You build up credits according to the amount of earnings you have each year, and the number of credits you need to qualify for disability benefits depends on your age when you become disabled.

For example, in 1988 workers earned one SSDI credit for each $470 of wages, up to a total of four credits with earnings of $1,840 or more. To qualify for SSDI upon becoming disabled (defined as an inability to work for at least a year), you must have earned six credits in the previous three years if under age 24, must have worked at least half the time between age 21 and the disability if age 24 through 31, have earned 20 credits if age 31 through 42, or have earned 20 credits plus at least one credit for each year above age 43. The average monthly benefit for an individual in 1988 was $508, and for a family it was $919.

If you have worked and paid into Social Security in the past and you or a dependent becomes disabled, check with your Social Security office to see if you qualify for SSDI.

Veteran's Benefits

If you completed a term of service in the U.S. military and received an honorary discharge, you and your family may be entitled to several types of benefits. These may include medical care at a Veteran's Administration (VA) hospital or medical center, a death benefit, and burial in a VA cemetery. You will need to show proof of your (or a family member's) military service to claim benefits. Contact your nearest VA office or hospital to see what benefits you might qualify for.

WHAT OTHER TYPES OF INSURANCE MIGHT A PERSON WITH EPILEPSY WANT OR NEED?

Depending on your financial status and whether you drive a car, you might want or need to purchase three other types of insurance.

Disability Insurance

If you are now working and want to be sure you or your family will have a source of income if you become disabled, you may want to purchase a disability policy. These provide a percentage of your current income for a certain number of months after your death or disability. Disability payments usually start three, six, or 12 months after the disability occurs. The sooner coverage starts, the higher the premium. For a young family, disability insurance may be more important than life insurance.

Liability Insurance

This type of insurance pays up to a certain amount if you are sued by someone for an injury that was somehow your fault or that you contributed to. This may be part of a homeowner's or automobile insurance policy. Even if you don't own a home or don't drive, you might want to purchase a liability policy, especially if you have a lot of assets that need to be protected from a possible lawsuit.

Automobile Insurance

Some states require that anyone who obtains a driver's license or owns an automobile must have automobile insurance. In other states, this is not required, but it is foolish to drive without insurance. An automobile policy usually covers several things, including collision coverage for repairs to your car and to other cars if involved in an accident with you, medical coverage for injuries suffered by you and others in an accident, and liability coverage in case you are sued for causing or being involved in an accident. For each part of the policy you can purchase options such as a low or high deductible amount on collision insurance, or a low or high ceiling on medical and liability coverage.

Automobile insurance rates are set according to the driver's age, the type of car, the accident rate in the area, how much the car is driven daily (to work or school), and the driver's driving record. People who have gotten several traffic tickets or been involved in several accidents may have to buy "risk" insurance, which may cost hundreds of dollars more per year than a regular policy. Carriers vary in their policy with respect to those who have epilepsy. Shop around!

Accident and Accidental Death Insurance

A very limited form of coverage is often available without a medical examination or history. These policies pay only for accidental death or accidental loss of a limb. For most people, they are too expensive for the coverage offered, but if you can't get a policy offering more complete coverage they are worth investigating.

Important: An individual, especially one with epilepsy, rarely can get as good coverage as that offered through an employer. If you have a job with good insurance, and lose it, take steps to convert it to individual coverage. New laws now make this possible in many cases, but it ordinarily must be done within 30 days of termination.

19

Protecting Your Legal Rights*

Not too many years ago, people with epilepsy were commonly denied many basic legal rights. They were sometimes treated as if they were insane, were sterilized against their will, were prevented from marrying and adopting children, were denied entry into the United States from other countries, and were seldom hired for any kind of meaningful work. Unfortunately, some of these ignorant practices still persist in some areas of the United States and other countries. However, in most areas, legal rights for people with epilepsy have improved greatly in recent decades, thanks mostly to the work of the Epilepsy Foundation of America (EFA) and its counterparts in other nations.

Even though a law prohibits a certain type of discrimination, it does not guarantee that everyone will follow it. And many laws allow a great deal of room for interpretation in any individual case. If you believe your legal rights are being denied, consider consulting a lawyer. Most lawyers will discuss your questions with you for a brief time for a fairly low fee (usually less than $50) and will then advise you on the legal merits of your case and how much it might cost to pursue it further. Also, many lawyers donate some of their time to working pro bono, which in Latin means "for good." If you have a low income, inquire about this through your state bar association (lawyer's professional association) or a law school.

This chapter provides general information on a few areas of legal rights about which our patients have frequent questions. However, laws often differ slightly among the states, and the details of certain laws change often. You may want to find out the exact details of current laws in your state by contacting your local EFA chapter or your state's office of the attorney general.

---

*This chapter is based on information contained in "The Legal Rights of Persons with Epilepsy" published by the EFA and updated regularly by its legal department.

HOW DO THE LEGAL RIGHTS OF PEOPLE WITH EPILEPSY DIFFER FROM THOSE OF OTHER PEOPLE?

Someday (soon, we hope) the answer to this question will be, "They don't." The reason this is not yet an accurate answer is that many poorly informed members of the government, private companies, and the public still don't realize that there is a great deal of variation among people with epilepsy. The EFA believes that people with epilepsy deserve to be evaluated as individuals, not according to the often erroneous assumptions that are made about everyone with the disorder.

In many areas, the fact that a person has epilepsy may lead to unfair treatment. Insurance, which we discussed in the previous chapter, is probably the biggest problem. However, this may change as more medical information becomes available on people with epilepsy, and as companies realize that there is a tremendous amount of variation in how epilepsy affects a person's life.

With regard to access to medical care, two general legal factors need to be understood: First, a doctor is under no obligation to *start* treating a person (for a seizure, for example), but once treatment has started it must be continued until the immediate problem has been controlled. Second, publicly owned medical centers must treat anyone who requires medical care. The quality of care provided at a county or city medical center is often as good or better than at private clinics or hospitals. Any patient who does not feel his medical care is adequate should discuss it with the doctors or nurses, and if still dissatisfied, request a second opinion if he can afford it. It is also possible to file a complaint with the institution's management, with the medical association in the area, or with a court of law.

Employment is another area that has improved quite a bit but that still has a long way to go. Every state now has some type of law prohibiting employers from refusing to hire people with disabilities, but some of these apply only to state employees. Most of these laws require that, to use a condition such as epilepsy as a reason not to hire someone, the employer must show that the person's epilepsy would make it impossible or unsafe for the person to do the job. The federal antidiscrimination law applies only to the federal government, and to employers who get federal funds or have federal contracts. See Chapter 17 for more information about employment. State laws are enforced by the state government; federal laws by the federal government.

People with epilepsy have a right to access to other types of services, such as public transportation, public programs, and any public place or private facility open to the public. If you feel that you have been denied access to any type of service or facility because of epilepsy, contact your local government or a lawyer. States have varying laws on these issues, but most prohibit discrimination in places of public accommodation, i.e., hotels, restaurants, etc.

WHAT RIGHTS DOES A PERSON WITH EPILEPSY HAVE IF ARRESTED OR SEARCHED?

Sometimes the police or public may think that a person having a seizure is drunk or under the influence of illegal drugs. The person may be arrested or detained because of this misperception. The best way to prevent this is to wear a medical identification bracelet or to carry it in a wallet or purse. Some states require police to search for medical identification if a person is unconscious or semiconscious.

Some states give the police and physicians the right to search for medical identification if a person is injured or disabled or behaves strangely in public. They also require that arrangements then quickly be made to contact a physician listed on the ID or to transport the person to a safe and appropriate place.

Another problem may occur if a person is carrying an antiepileptic medication in a nonprescription container. This medication may be taken away for testing, possibly causing the person to have a seizure. Arrested persons might avoid these problems by telling police about their medical condition and asking them to contact the physician who prescribed the medication. You should carry medication in the prescription container if practical, or ask the pharmacist for a second, smaller, labeled container. You can also carry a copy of the prescription with you.

HOW DOES EPILEPSY AFFECT ADOPTION OR CHILD CUSTODY RIGHTS?

Epilepsy may become a consideration in an adoption or child custody proceeding for two reasons: (1) if an adult has epilepsy it might be one factor that is considered in evaluating his ability to be an adequate parent, and (2) it is more difficult to find adoptive homes for children with epilepsy.

No state law specifically cites epilepsy as a factor in determining an adult's fitness to be a parent. The main factor in any adoption or custody hearing is to provide for the child's best interests. This includes making sure that the prospective parents are able to provide for the child's emotional and physical needs. The health of a parent may become an issue in this, but epilepsy is not an absolute disqualifier. Courts must consider the individual's ability to conduct his or her life and to care for a child.

Some children with epilepsy are severely disabled and are therefore harder to place for adoption. State and federal adoption assistance programs provide financial assistance to parents who adopt such "hard to place" children. Only one state, California, still has a law that allows adoptive parents to petition to annul an adoption if, within five years of the adoption, the child has symptoms of a severe disability that existed without their knowledge before the adoption.

WHAT EDUCATIONAL RIGHTS DO PEOPLE WITH EPILEPSY HAVE?

The Education for All Handicapped Children Act (P.L. 94-142) provides that handicapped children are entitled to a free, appropriate, public education. States must identify and provide specially trained professionals to evaluate children in need of special services. Epilepsy is included as a potential reason for eligibility, but it must be shown that the child's ability or performance in school is adversely affected by the disorder. Individual instruction provided early and by a teacher trained to help overcome learning disabilities related to epilepsy can help a child achieve his maximum educational potential.

An important part of this federal law requires that, wherever possible, handicapped children have access to an education with children who are not handicapped. This helps children with epilepsy adjust to the disorder and develop good self-esteem. But it also helps teachers and other children understand and accept disabilities and disorders such as epilepsy.

Every child is entitled to a free public education through high school. Higher education is not free, but federal law requires that admission procedures be fair. Very few state colleges and universities even ask if a prospective student has epilepsy. Those that ask about epilepsy or other medical conditions report that this information is used to identify medical needs of the students. The EFA believes that such information should be provided voluntarily if at all, and must be kept confidential and not used as a basis to deny admission. Students with epilepsy may want to provide relevant information to the student health service in case they need assistance while at school. Also, some colleges have a student epilepsy support group that can help overcome problems that might be encountered on campus.

WHAT ARE THE LEGAL RIGHTS OF INMATES IN CORRECTIONAL FACILITIES?

Epilepsy is one of the more common chronic illnesses of people in prison. Studies show that the prevalence rate of epilepsy among people in prisons and jails is approximately three times greater than in the general population. Earlier theories that attributed this to a connection between epilepsy and a tendency toward violence have been rejected. Rather, the higher incidence of epilepsy among prisoners is attributed to sociological factors. Three such factors have been identified. First, due to the stigma associated with epilepsy and society's frequent rejection of persons with the condition, some people with epilepsy have difficulty adjusting socially. This may result in an increased incidence of hostile behavior. Second, people who are involved in criminal activity are more likely to have been beaten up and to be involved in alcohol abuse. They are, therefore, more likely to develop epilepsy from head injury or alcohol abuse or withdrawal. Finally, people with epilepsy of lower socioeconomic status are more likely to be imprisoned for their acts.

Several professional health organizations have identified a lack of adequate medical care for inmates with epilepsy and other chronic health problems. The American Medical Association has published a recommended outline for an epilepsy treatment program in correctional institutions and has identified minimum levels of care. These include a careful medical screening for epilepsy in incoming inmates, contacting a physician or medical facility to prepare an organized treatment plan with periodic examinations, and a training program to help staff administer medications and provide first aid for seizures.

Prisoners who are denied adequate medical care should consult an attorney about the legal options open to them. A successful lawsuit will usually require proof of intentional mistreatment or deliberate neglect of a serious medical need, with resultant serious harm.

CAN A PERSON WITH EPILEPSY BE COMMITTED INVOLUNTARILY TO A MENTAL HEALTH FACILITY?

No state allows commitment based solely on a person's epilepsy, and most states' involuntary commitment laws are limited to people who are mentally ill or mentally retarded. Even in these cases, it must usually be shown that the person is a danger to himself or others, or is incapable of self-care. The EFA does not believe that epilepsy is a reason to take an individual's freedom away, and that even when epilepsy is accompanied by mental illness or mental retardation, involuntary commitment should be a last resort. If commitment is necessary, every effort should be made to protect the rights of the person and to guarantee continuing medical treatment according to accepted standards.

Several states allow parents or guardians of a person with epilepsy to admit that person temporarily to a respite facility, even if the person with epilepsy does not want to stay there. The time limit for this involuntary respite care ranges from 21 to 30 days.

IS IT LEGAL TO DISCRIMINATE AGAINST PEOPLE WITH EPILEPSY IN HOUSING, LENDING, OR PUBLIC SERVICES?

According to the EFA, a majority of the states prohibit discrimination in housing based on handicaps such as epilepsy. Some states prohibit such discrimination in lending agreements and credit transactions. Some states have laws against denying handicapped persons access to public transportation. These laws vary widely, and obviously they are less than ideal protection for the rights of people with epilepsy and others with handicaps.

The EFA supports the extension of state civil rights laws to include the handicapped, and also supports the passage of a comprehensive federal law—The Americans with Disabilities Act. In states where laws do not give people with epilepsy equal access to housing, credit, and public services, pressure should be brought on public officials and owners of private facilities serving the public. The type of legal action that can be taken under current laws varies from state to state, and in some cases federal law may offer protections. It is a good idea to contact a lawyer or the state human rights commission if you feel you have been discriminated against in any of these areas.

DO PEOPLE WITH EPILEPSY HAVE A RIGHT TO DRIVE?

No one in the United States has a *right* to drive. Operating a motor vehicle is a privilege that must be earned and qualified for through existing state laws that are intended to protect the public as much as possible from the potential dangers involved. Every state regulates the driving eligibility of people with certain medical conditions. Most require that a person with epilepsy be seizure-free for a certain amount of time and submit a physician's evaluation of their ability to drive safely. Some states require periodic reports from the person's physician. Check with your state's Department of Motor Vehicles about current requirements.

Some states are starting to allow more individual evaluation in granting driver's licenses to people with epilepsy. Exceptions are being allowed for people who have only nighttime seizures, for those who have enough of a warning of a seizure (aura) to stop a car, and for those who have a seizure as a result of a physician's change in their medication. Restricted licenses may be available that allow a person with epilepsy to drive to and from work, within a certain distance from home, or in an emergency.

The EFA supports the establishment of medical advisory boards, with at least one neurologist member experienced in epilepsy, to advise states on licensing laws and to mediate requests for driving privileges. Many states have already established such a board. They are finding that this type of review process can be much fairer in reviewing individual situations and granting driving privileges while protecting the public's safety.

HOW CAN I HELP PROTECT AND EXTEND THE RIGHTS OF PEOPLE WITH EPILEPSY?

Discrimination against people with epilepsy is still a major problem in our society, sometimes causing more problems than the disorder itself. By knowing the laws in your area and by being willing to take whatever steps necessary to protect the rights of people with epilepsy and other handicaps, you can make major contributions. Support the efforts of and contribute in whatever way you can to national, state, and local offices of the EFA. By doing these things, you can both benefit from and help continue the progress that has been made in recent years.

20

Resources: Here's Where to Turn When You Need Help

Florence Gray

Everyone needs help from others at times. Most people don't rely entirely on their own skills and abilities to get through life successfully. They know whom to ask for information and where to go to get the things they need to live well. The organizations listed in this chapter are especially good at helping people live well with epilepsy. Contact them for general information, advice, support, health care, and to find out what services are available in your area.

ADVOCACY AND ASSISTANCE FOR PEOPLE WITH EPILEPSY

The Epilepsy Foundation of America (EFA) (4351 Garden City Drive, Landover, MD 20785; 301-459-3700; toll-free, 1-800-EFA-1000) is the only national, charitable, nonprofit voluntary agency in the United States specifically dedicated to the welfare of people with epilepsy. Approximately 100 local organizations around the country are affiliated with the EFA. If you don't know the phone number or address of your nearest affiliate, call the toll-free national number.

The EFA national office publishes information and presents educational programs on epilepsy, works with lawmakers to encourage the passage of laws that treat people with epilepsy fairly, and supports epilepsy research. EFA also publishes a monthly newsletter called *National Spokesman*.

State and local EFA affiliates are usually United Way agencies and offer a range of services and programs depending on the support they receive. Programs may include:

- Information and referral services
- School Alert programs to improve the school environment for children with epilepsy
- Self-help groups and parent groups

- Recreational and education programs for young people with epilepsy
- Community education, especially during November, which is National Epilepsy Month
- Educational programs for health-care professionals
- Community residences for people with epilepsy who need some help in order to live independently
- Counseling for people with epilepsy and their families
- Advocacy for those who are being discriminated against because of epilepsy
- Job finding and employer educational programs (Training and Placement Service).

HEALTH CARE FOR PEOPLE WITH EPILEPSY

Comprehensive Epilepsy Programs (CEPs)

The development of programs specifically designed for and dedicated to treating and studying epilepsy—CEPs—was spurred by a policy statement from the National Institute for Neurological Disorders and Stroke (NINDS), a part of the National Institutes of Health (NIH). This statement noted in part that "epilepsy is a complicated, chronic disorder and should be treated in a comprehensive way."

Money from the NIH research budget was provided in 1975 to start CEPs in Minnesota (MINCEP Epilepsy Care, P.A.), Virginia (University of Virginia Comprehensive Epilepsy Program), and Oregon (Comprehensive Epilepsy Center of Oregon). In 1976, NIH funds were provided for CEPs in Augusta (Georgia Comprehensive Epilepsy Program), and Seattle (Regional Epilepsy Program). In 1980, a CEP opened in Los Angeles (UCLA Urban Comprehensive Epilepsy Program). The CEPs were created to provide the best care for people with epilepsy; to serve as a laboratory for multidisciplinary research; to educate doctors, nurses, and other caregivers; and to organize community services.

At the end of 1988, only the CEPs in Minnesota, Seattle, and Los Angeles continued to receive NIH funding. This lack of support has reduced services or closed some of the other CEPs. Yet, they have proven and some continue to demonstrate the validity of a comprehensive, multidisciplinary approach. They are helping to improve seizure control in many patients with difficult seizures, they are improving the lives of individuals with epilepsy and their families, and they are greatly expanding knowledge of the clinical treatment of epilepsy.

If you continue to have seizures or are experiencing side-effects that make it difficult for you to think or function in daily life, discuss the problem with your doctor or obtain a neurologist's opinion. If your seizure control or alertness still does not improve, seek help at a CEP if there is one in your region. If there is not, contact the national EFA or the local affiliate for a referral to a reputable program near you. Or you can call the National Association of Epilepsy Centers (612-331-4477), which is trying to improve access to and the quality of care offered by epilepsy treatment programs.

PUBLICATIONS AND AUDIOVISUAL MATERIALS ON EPILEPSY

The following centers are active in producing educational materials on epilepsy. Some publications may be free, but others must be purchased; audiovisual materials usually can be either rented or purchased. Contact them for a current catalogue of their offerings.

Epilepsy Foundation of America
4351 Garden City Drive
Landover, MD 20785
301-459-3700; toll-free, 1-800-EFA-1000

MINCEP Epilepsy Care, P.A.
2701 University Avenue, S.E.
Suite 106
Minneapolis, MN 55414
612-627-4477

Comprehensive Epilepsy Program
Bowman Gray School of Medicine
Winston-Salem, NC 27103
1-800-642-0500 (toll-free in North Carolina)

LEGAL ASSISTANCE AND INFORMATION FOR PEOPLE WITH DISABILITIES

Administration on Developmental Disabilities (ADD)

Write to Room 340E, Hubert H. Humphrey Building, 200 Independence Avenue, S.W., Washington, D.C. 20201 for the location of the ADD office nearest you, which can provide specialized help and information on laws and services for people with disabling medical conditions.

Epilepsy Foundation of America

The EFA publishes a comprehensive, up-to-date, loose-leaf binder on federal and state laws pertaining to epilepsy. A pamphlet on the legal rights of people with epilepsy is also available. (See address and phone earlier in chapter.)

Camps for Children and Teens with Epilepsy

A child whose seizures are well-controlled can probably safely attend any well-supervised, reputable camp for children (see Chapter 12 for a discussion of how and why to choose a camp). Children whose seizures are not necessarily well-controlled, or who want to learn more about epilepsy and share experiences with other children with the disorder, may benefit greatly from a camp specifically for children with epilepsy. These camps also may offer special programs for teens with epilepsy, as well as an opportunity for the teen to be a counselor for children with epilepsy.

The camps listed in Table 20-1 have provided information to the EFA about their benefits for children with epilepsy. Parents should contact the camp director for complete information on the camp's medical staff, educational program, recreational activities, facilities, safety procedures, length and dates, cost, and the age range and medical condition of youth accepted. Parents and their children also may want to attend an orientation meeting and open house at the camp before deciding whether to attend.

HELP FOR PARENTS OF CHILDREN WITH CHRONIC DISORDERS OR DISABILITIES

The National Network of Parent Centers, Inc.

This is a national network of organizations called Technical Assistance for Parent Programs (TAPP). It is funded by the U.S. Department of Education, Office of Special Education and Rehabilitative Services. TAPP programs provide training and information to parents of handicapped children. They have created an environment in which experienced, knowledgeable parents can help other parents. To find the TAPP in your area, contact the national office or the office for your region.

National Office: Federation for Children with Special Needs, 312 Stuart Street, Boston, MA 02116; 617-482-2915.

Northeast Regional Center: New Hampshire Parent Information Center, P.O. Box 1422, Concord, NH 03301; 603-224-7005 (serves New Hampshire, Maine, Vermont, Connecticut, New York, Rhode Island,

Table 20-1. *Camps for Children with Epilepsy*

State	Camp and sponsor	Length	Contact
California	LACES camp, Los Angeles County Epilepsy Society	Weekend	Catalina Rofloc 213-382-7337
Florida	S.E. Florida Everglades Conservation Youth Camp, Florida Epilepsy Foundation	Week	Linda Swanson 904-378-6737
Georgia	Camp Toccoa Georgia Chapter, EFA	Week	Dorothy Frazier 404-527-7155
Illinois	Epilepsy Summer Retreat	Weekend	Epilepsy Association of SW Illinois 618-236-2181
Minnesota	Camp Oz, EF of Minnesota–MINCEP Epilepsy Care, P.A., and Gillette Children's Hospital	Week	Deb McNally 612-627-4477
Pennsylvania	Camp "R," EF of Western Pennsylvania	Week	Lee Phillips (No phone given)
Tennessee	Camp Lakewood, EF of Greater Chattanooga	Week	Theresa Ingram 615-756-1771
Texas	YMCA Camp Carter, Fort Worth-Tarrant County EA	Week	Louann Levis 817-336-8693
Washington	Camp Sealth-Campfire	Week	Epilepsy Association of Western Washington 206-523-2551
Wisconsin	Phantom Lake Camp, Epilepsy Center, South Central	Week	Dan Miller 608-257-5759

Massachusetts, Pennsylvania, New Jersey, Delaware, Maryland, Puerto Rico, and Washington, D.C.).

West Regional Center: Washington State PAVE, 1010 South "I" Street, Tacoma, WA 98405; 206-272-7804 (serves Washington, Montana, Wyoming, Idaho, Oregon, Alaska, Hawaii, Utah, California, Texas, New Mexico, Arizona, Nevada, Department of Defense Dependents' Schools (DODDS), and The American Territories).

Midwest Regional Center: PACER Center, Inc., 4826 Chicago Avenue, Minneapolis, MN 55417; 612-827-2966 (serves Wisconsin, Michigan, Ohio, Indiana, Iowa, Illinois, Kentucky, Missouri, Kansas, Nebraska, Minnesota, North Dakota, South Dakota, and Colorado).

South Regional Center: PEP, Georgia ARC, 1851 Ram Runway, No. 104, College Park, GA 30337; 404-761-2745 (serves Georgia, Arkansas, Louisiana, Mississippi, Alabama, Florida, South Carolina, Tennessee, Virginia, West Virginia, and Oklahoma).

The following organizations have received funding from the Division of Maternal and Child Health, U.S. Public Health Service, to help parents and professionals improve families' ability to provide care for children with special health-care needs. They can provide audiovisual materials, publications, technical assistance, and referral to programs in your area.

Association for the Care of Children's Health (ACCH)
3615 Wisconsin Avenue, N.W.
Washington, D.C. 20016
202-244-1801

An association of professionals and parents that provides written and audiovisual materials as well as consultation services to help people take a family-centered approach to caring for children with special health needs.

Federation for Children with Special Needs
312 Stuart Street
Boston, MA 02116
617-482-2915

Administers the Collaboration Among Parents and (Health) Professionals (CAPP) project. This project encourages parent involvment in the health care of their children with chronic illness or disability, and it promotes partnerships between parents and health-care professionals.

National Maternal and Child Health Resource Center
College of Law Building
The University of Iowa
Iowa City, IA 52242
319-335-9046

Provides information, assistance, and training materials to promote the improvement and expansion of maternal and child health services, including services for children with special health-care needs.

Community Resources and Social Services

Most cities, counties, and states support an array of social services that provide financial, educational, vocational, legal, residential, counseling, and transportation needs. It may seem confusing to try to find the services in your area and to gain access to them, but be persistent. If you aren't sure where to go for help or don't get the help you need, ask for help from a social worker or from your local EFA affiliate.

Table 20-2 lists general services that are available in most areas and tells how to find each service. This table has been taken from: *Family Dynamics: Understanding and Helping Your Family Function in a More Positive Way,* a book by Judy L. Antonello, published in 1982 by Family Psychological Services.

Table 20-2. *Community Resource List for Parents*

Service needed	Common provider agency	How usually listed in local directory	Possible eligibility requirements
Financial assistance			
Aid to families with dependent children (AFDC)	County Welfare Department	Under *County* and provider name	Resident of county, single parent or family with child(ren) usually under 19 in school
General assistance (GA)	County Welfare Department	Under *County* and provider name	Resident of county unable to work, disabled, a displaced homemaker
General assistance medical care (GAMC)	County Welfare Department	Under *County* and provider name	Resident of county unable to pay for medical care
Medical assistance (MA)	Usually State Department of Public Welfare administered by the county	Under *County* and provider name	Resident of county unable to pay for medical care
Social Security benefits	Social Security Administration	Under *U.S.* and provider name	Disabled child or adult
Supplemental Security Income (SSI)	Social Security Administration	Under *U.S.* and provider name	

Service needed	Common provider agency	How usually listed in local directory	Possible eligibility requirements
Funds for medical care and equipment for children with handicaps	State Department of Health Services for Children with Handicaps or Crippled Children's Service	Under *State* and provider name	Resident of State under 21 and handicapping conditions
Food stamps	Usually administered by the County Welfare Department	Under *County* and provider name	Resident of county and income requirement for household
Employment, vocational and educational			
Employment	State Office Economic Security Department	Under *State* and provider name; yellow pages: *employment agency*	Working age
Vocational assessment training and job placement for disabled individuals	State Offices Economic Security Division of Vocational Rehabilitation	Under *State* and provider name	Working age, disabled to degree, limits job opportunities
Education	State Department of Education and local public school district	Under *State* and provider name; also local public school district	
Home support services			
Public health nursing	State Department of Health	Under *State* and provider name	Varies
Homemaker/ housekeeping services	County Department of Welfare	Under *County* and provider name	
Chore services	County Department of Welfare	Under *County* and provider name	
Home health aid/ nurse	Private agencies and requests thru County Welfare Social Services	Under *County*; yellow pages: *nurses*	

Service needed	Common provider agency	How usually listed in local directory	Possible eligibility requirements
Babysitting	Varies	Under yellow pages: *Daycare;* also contact *County* Welfare Department (Social Service) for list of licensed daycare	
Transportation	County Department Welfare Volunteer Service, State Department of Public Transportation, Local Public Transit, Private Ambulance Medical Transportation Service	Under *County* and provider name, *State* and provider name; yellow pages: *buses, taxis, ambulance service*	
Legal services	County Bar Association, County Attorney's Office, Public Defender, Legal Aid Societies	Under *County* and provider name; also yellow pages: *attorney referral service* and *attorneys*	Varies
Child protection services (abuse and neglect)	County Welfare Department Child Protection Unit	Under *County* and provider name	Usually any child being abused or neglected
Child or adult out-of-home placement	County Welfare Department Placement Unit	Under *County* and provider name	Varies
Respite care	County Welfare Department Placement Unit or special project in community	Under *County* and provider name	Varies

Service needed	Common provider agency	How usually listed in local directory	Possible eligibility requirements
Counseling services			
Individual	Community Mental Health Centers, private agencies and individuals, county social services	Under *County community services, mental health, County Welfare Social Services,* yellow pages for *psychologist, psychiatrist, social workers* (and related professional associations), *child guidance, marriage and family counseling*	Varies
Marital/couple	Community Mental Health Centers, private agencies and individuals, county social service	Same as above	Varies
Family	Community Mental Health Centers, private agencies and individuals, county social service	Same as above	Varies
Group counseling service	Same as above	Same as above	Varies
Chemical dependency	Local hospital programs, specific programs set up for chemical dependency treatment, Alcoholics Anonymous, Alanon, Alateen	Under yellow pages: *alcoholism information and treatment centers* and *drug abuse and addiction information centers* and *treatment centers*	Chemically dependent; other requirements vary

Service needed	Common provider agency	How usually listed in local directory	Possible eligibility requirements
Support and self-help groups	Varies	Under yellow pages: *associations*; check problem area in white pages, e.g., Spina Bifida Association	Usually open to anyone interested
Housing Low-to-moderate income for families, disabled, elderly	Housing and Redevelopment Authority, American Red Cross	Under *City* and *Township* or *County* and provider name; *American Red Cross* in white pages	Families, disabled, and elderly (usually have income eligibility requirements)
Adoption	State Department of Public Welfare Adoption Unit and County Department of Welfare, also Community Family Service Agencies	Under *State* and provider home, *County* and provider name. Yellow pages under *adoption agency*	Varies

21

Research: Hope for Today and the Future

Ilo E. Leppik, M.D., and Robert J. Gumnit, M.D.

We live in an exciting time of scientific advances. Much new knowledge has been gained about the structures within the brain and their functions. However, there is still a long way to go before we understand how the brain stores and processes information, how it directs the many functions of the body, and what goes wrong when a seizure occurs. Scientists are piecing together this information in many types of research. This chapter describes some of the research areas that show the most promise for improving the lives of people with epilepsy.

WHAT ARE THE DIFFERENT TYPES OF RESEARCH?

The word "research" brings to mind a scientist in a laboratory. Actually, laboratory science is only one type of research. Several other areas of research are necessary to bring laboratory discoveries to the point where they can be useful to people. We will discuss three general areas of research: basic science, developmental research, and clinical research.

Basic Science

This is the popular image of the scientist in a laboratory, surrounded by glass beakers and complicated equipment. Although this is what most people see in their mind's eye when they think of research, it is the least understood area of research. The reason it is called basic science is because its purpose is to study biological systems and to try to understand basic facts about life.

Basic science is difficult for most people to understand because it has become very complex. Scientists must specialize in one area of biology, and they must focus their efforts on answering very specific questions about one area of that specialty.

For example, a scientist who studies the nervous system is called a neuroscientist. But the nervous system is so complex that no one neuroscientist could ever attempt to study the entire nervous system. One neuroscientist might focus on the type of nerve cells that connect the retina of the eye to the part of the brain responsible for sight, while another studies the type of nerve cells that are involved in certain kinds of seizures. As each scientist answers a specific question about the nervous system, he or she writes an article for publication in a research journal, usually one devoted to neuroscience research. Journals and scientific meetings enable neuroscientists to share their discoveries and to learn from the successes and mistakes of other scientists.

Money to support basic research comes mostly from the National Institutes of Health (NIH), in Bethesda, Maryland, which is funded by taxpayers' money distributed by Congress. Funds for neuroscience research come from a branch of the NIH called the National Institute of Neurological Disorders and Stroke. Funding for basic research is used to buy laboratory equipment and animals, and to pay for the thousands of experiments needed to answer one scientific question. The discoveries made by a basic researcher might help explain a disorder such as epilepsy, but that is not the specific purpose of this stage of research.

The purpose of basic science is to explain how living things function, not to try to fix things that have gone wrong. Most of the really important scientific breakthroughs have occurred because a scientist was studying the function of a very small part of a living system and discovered a basic rule about how that system is organized or functions. This basic understanding then provides a clue for a scientist working in the next area of research—developmental research.

Developmental Research

Scientists working in this area of research are interested in developing equipment, drugs, or animal models that can be used to study or treat human diseases and disorders. They use the information provided by basic research as a place to start. The funds for this type of research come mostly from the NIH and from private companies that might benefit from the new development.

The development of new scientific and medical equipment has greatly improved the ability of scientists to study the nervous system in the laboratory and in the clinic. Two areas that have advanced most drastically are new types of microscopes and new types of medical imaging devices.

Scientists have developed several new types of microscopes that enable them to see very tiny structures within cells. These are electron microscopes (newer versions are called scanning tunneling microscopes and the atomic force microscope) because they used electrons rather than light to create a picture of cells. Standard light microscopes can reveal groups of cells and some detail of larger cells, but they are limited by the fairly long wavelength of light. Electrons have shorter wavelengths and can therefore reveal smaller features of cells. Electron microscopes greatly increased scientists' knowledge about what is inside cells such as neurons. But to view something on an electron microscope, it must be sliced very thin and treated with chemicals. This is fine for seeing very small details, but it doesn't allow the scientist to tell how those structures function in the cell.

A new type of microscope has recently been developed that enables scientists to see cell structures that are still alive and functioning. Called a confocal laser scanning microscope, it uses very intense laser light to create thousands of pictures of relatively thick slices of tissue. The pictures are sent to a computer that builds them into one composite picture of the structures within the tissue. The computer also enables the scientist to rotate the picture, to see what the structures look like from every angle. Laser microscopes are just beginning to be used to study how neurons function, but scientists expect this new device to greatly expand knowledge about the nervous system, and possibly about what goes wrong in the brains of people with epilepsy.

Another field that has advanced very rapidly in the past decade is neuroradiology—the taking of pictures of the brain and the rest of the nervous system. Neurologists used to have to rely on X-rays or gamma rays to take pictures of the head, spine, and extremities. X-rays reveal bones very well, but they don't show soft tissue such as the brain or nerves in any detail.

This changed when CT (computed tomography) devices were developed about 15 years ago. And then, about five years ago, MRI (magnetic resonance imaging) devices were developed. MRI uses a different type of energy to produce pictures of the brain (see Chapter 6). CT uses conventional X-rays; MRI uses magnetic energy. MRI is now the preferred method of diagnosing tumors and other abnormal structures in the nervous system.

CT and MRI were developed by basic researchers in the area of physics. These physicists studied how atomic structures such as electrons, positrons, neutrons, and photons pass through structures and are affected by various forms of energy. Their discoveries were used by other scientists to develop computerized "cameras" that could recreate the physical structures they passed through. Now a new form of imaging device called SPECT (single-proton emission computed tomography) and PET (positron emission tomography) has been developed by physicists and developmental researchers.

The primary purpose of SPECT and PET is not to show the structures of the brain, but rather to show what is happening within those structures. Different intensity of chemical reactions shows up as different colors on a computer monitor. This enables scientists to compare normal scans to those of a person with epilepsy, for example, and to see if there are any differences in the way the person's brain is functioning. PET is far more expensive than SPECT, and rapid developments are taking place in both.

Another way that basic scientists stimulate developmental research is by explaining exactly how something works in a living system. This then suggests ways to study what goes wrong in a disease or disorder, and to try to fix it. For example, a basic scientist may discover that the gap between neurons where messages are exchanged—the synapse—requires a certain electrochemical mixture in order to function efficiently. This scientist may then attempt to try other chemicals and electrical stimuli to see how they affect the exchange of messages. Or the basic scientist may pass the discovery on to another scientist who is interested in developing drugs that block or improve the exchange of messages at synapses involved in seizures.

In fact, the study of synapses is a major area of research that supplies clues to the causes and treatment of epilepsy. Scientists are trying to understand how nerve cells in the brain communicate with each other by exchanging electrochemical messages at synapses. When a person has epilepsy, this system sometimes becomes overloaded. Millions of neurons get out of control and begin exchanging erroneous electrochemical messages that cause the person to behave in the ways characteristic of a certain type of seizure.

The developmental researcher may take the new knowledge about synapses and try to develop a substance that will stabilize the exchange of electrochemical messages. Some of this work can be done with isolated neurons in laboratory cultures. But a major portion must be done in living animals—mostly mice and rats. The most significant developmental research in the past 15 years has been the selective breeding of animal models for epilepsy. Scientists have identified types of mice and rats that have seizures when given a certain chemical or other stimulus. By breeding these animals, the scientists have made available thousands of animal models that can be used to test chemical compounds designed to block epileptic seizures.

The availability of animal models for epilepsy now makes it possible to test thousands of compounds every year in the laboratory. Each compound is given to an animal to see if it can block a seizure. If it can, other tests are done on the animal to see if it can still function and be healthy when taking an effective dose of the seizure-preventing compound. Thanks to the excellent animal models and testing procedures developed by laboratory scientists, each trial compound can be tested in less than a week.

If a compound appears to be effective in this first phase of animal testing, it is then tested in other animals to see if it is harmful in any way. Different amounts and ways of administering the drug may also be tested. Then, after as much information as possible has been gained from animal research, the Food and Drug Administration reviews an application from the developers and decides whether to approve testing the compound in humans, which is called clinical research.

Why is animal research still necessary?

Before we discuss clinical research, it is important to understand why animal research is very necessary. Throughout the history of medical research, people have wrestled with the ethics of using animals to advance human knowledge. Groups once known as antivivisectionists have been active since the 19th century, opposing the use of animals in scientific education and research.

One of the favored tactics of animal rights groups is to say that animal research has not resulted in any medical gains in the past. They know that most people don't receive information about the history of medicine in school or in the mass media. In fact, *without animal research, there would be no vaccine for polio or any other infectious disease, people with insulin-dependent diabetes would die within months because insulin would not be available, there would be no open heart surgery or any other complicated surgical procedure, and people with epilepsy would have uncontrollable seizures because there would be no new antiepileptic medications.*

Despite these advances—and many more—and the millions of people suffering the enormous toll of diseases not yet conquered, animal rights groups argue that animal research should be restricted or stopped. They assert that medical science and education should be able to proceed using cell cultures or computer simulations of biological systems. This is simply not true.

Another charge of animal rights organizations is to assert that medical researchers receive funding for projects that involve torturing animals for no clear research purpose. This tactic takes advantage of the public's lack of information about the competitiveness of research grants and the very strict guidelines that must be followed. The NIH has set up very strict guidelines for reviewing proposals for animal research, and for making sure that the research is carried out with a minimum of distress to the animals.

In addition, each university or research organization must have an animal research committee that is made up of some members of the outside community, often the local animal humane society representative. This committee approves applications and oversees animal research and education laboratories, making sure that repetitive or unnecessary research is not being done, and that all possible steps are taken to prevent animals from suffering. The U.S. Department of Agriculture assists the NIH in holding surprise inspections of these facilities to make sure rules about cage sizes, cleanliness, and animal care are being strictly adhered to.

Animal rights activists and medical researchers actually share a common goal: achieving a world without animal research. However, animal rights activists want to have that world right now, at the expense of the millions of people affected by diseases and disorders. Medical researchers and educators would also like to do away with the need for animals, because they do not like to hurt or kill. Medical researchers understand how little we really know about living systems, and they therefore appreciate how important animals will be for a very long time to come.

If Congress were to outlaw animal research, as animal rights activists continue to suggest, not only medical research but medical education as well would stop. Our medical schools would graduate doctors who had never gone beyond a textbook or computer in learning living anatomy and physiology. Also, medical treatments would be frozen in time. Can you imagine going in for a new type of surgery that has never been tried on a living thing? Can you imagine taking a medication that has not been tested on animals and whose toxicity and long-term effects are therefore unknown? The fact is that no pharmaceutical company would market such a drug, and no medical school would graduate such a surgeon.

In other words, we would live in a world without new medications and treatments for diseases such as heart disease, cancer, diabetes, and epilepsy.

Polls continue to show that 75–85% of the U.S. public understands the importance of animal research and believes that it should continue. If you agree, it is important that you contact your representatives in Congress and in your state legislature, and that you support your local medical school or research institution. And, if you have a chance, take the time to provide some accurate information in response to the wishful thinking and misinformation spread by animal rights organizations.

Clinical Research

After animal research has proved that a compound or treatment is effective and safe—at least in animals as close to humans as possible—the FDA can approve clinical testing. There are several steps involved in testing any new medication or treatment on humans.

Let's assume that the FDA has approved human testing of a potential antiepileptic medication. The first step is very limited testing of the drug on healthy people who do not have epilepsy. This step involves a relatively small number of people who are monitored closely to see if the new treatment has any unexpected side-effects or affects humans differently than it did animals. If this step is successful, the FDA approves the next step, which is testing on people whose seizures are not well controlled by any other medication. This is usually interpreted to be people who have four or more seizures per month.

There are many different procedures for testing a potential antiepileptic medication, but at this time all initial testing must be done on people who are 18 years or older. Most initial testing is done in the hospital, to allow neurologists to closely monitor the effectiveness and safety of the medication. Pharmacists and clinical nurses are also often involved in monitoring the patient's therapy and keeping blood levels of the experimental medication at desired levels.

If inpatient testing shows that the medication is safe and effective, the FDA can approve outpatient testing in people who meet the strictly defined indications of the clinical research project. For example, this might be males with epilepsy who are between 18 and 40 years old—the FDA wants to prevent problems in women who may become pregnant and in children and older people. These limited clinical tests may last for two or three years. Then, depending on how effective and safe the medication is shown to be, the FDA may approve it for use in other groups of people with epilepsy, including women and children.

If all goes well in clinical testing, the FDA will grant marketing rights giving the pharmaceutical company authorization to market the medication for the purpose for which it has been proved effective and safe. Physicians can then prescribe it according to their professional judgment about whether it will help control a person's seizures. All serious side-effects must be reported to the FDA to allow ongoing monitoring and reporting of the medication's safety.

The process that starts with testing a new compound in animals and sometimes results in its approval as a medication for sale to humans usually takes anywhere from five to 10 years. This seems too long for people with the disease or disorder it is intended to treat, especially if it is a fatal disease such as AIDS. The FDA has shortened the time necessary to approve human use of AIDS drugs, and there may be similar improvements in efficiency with other medications.

There is a big difference between greater efficiency and reduced caution, however. No one wants to see new drugs rushed onto the market before anyone knows how they will affect certain groups of people over the many years that they will be used.

HOW CAN I HELP PROMOTE EPILEPSY RESEARCH?

There are many ways to contribute to epilepsy research. The most obvious is by donating money for neuroscience or epilepsy studies at your local research institution, or for clinical research at an epilepsy center. You can also write letters or visit with your representatives in national and state governments to make sure they understand the importance of funding epilepsy research. You can combine your efforts with others by supporting the national research programs of the EFA.

If you have epilepsy and your seizures are not well controlled, you may be asked by your doctor or nurse to consider participating in a clinical research program. Make sure you understand what will be required of you throughout the project. Your first consideration should be whether the project might help improve your epilepsy control and general well-being. Many people also benefit from the feeling that they are helping other people with epilepsy. If you decide to participate, it is very important that you follow directions exactly so that the information gained is as accurate as possible and as helpful to you and others as possible.

Healthy relatives of people with epilepsy or concerned citizens can also support epilepsy research through advocacy or monetary contributions, or by volunteering for initial testing of FDA-approved experimental medications. And, finally, we can all support all types of medical research by helping to educate our friends, neighbors, and children about the reasons animal research is necessary, and about the tremendous gains that are being made toward the day when epilepsy and other disorders and diseases will be footnotes in history.

INDEX

Disability insurance, 133
Discrimination. *See* Legal rights
Divalproex (Depakote), 32
  in breast milk, 115
Dizziness, anticonvulsants, 34
Doctor–patient relationship, satisfaction
  with, 23–24
Driving, automobile, 85,86,140–141
Drugs, illegal, 91–92
Dudley, Dr. Benjamin, 41

Education, 81–83
  legal rights, 138
Education of All Handicapped Children
  Act (P.L. 94–192), 81
EEG
  diagnosis, 27,29–30
    electrodes, 27
  epilepsy and violence, 101
  infants, seizures in, 54–55,57,59
  pre-surgical, 44
  seizure, 7,9,10
  surgical treatment, 41
    post-surgical monitoring, 46
Electrodes, EEG, 27
Electron microscopes, 154–155
Employment, 149
  legal rights, 119–120,136
Epilepsy
  advocacy groups, 142–143; *see also*
    Epilepsy Foundation of America
  audiovisual materials, 144
  causes, 11–12
  definition, 2,6–8
    vs. seizure disorder, 61–62
  diagnosis, first reactions to, 1–2
  family role in treatment, 3
  patient feelings about, 3–4
  prevalence, U.S., 2
  publications on, 144
  public education, 53
  treatment, 12–14
  types, 8–9
  uncontrolled, 14
  violence and, no link, 101,139
  see also Seizure(s); *specific aspects*
Epilepsy Foundation of America (EFA),
  18–20,49,83,120,121,129,142–144,
  148,160
  legal rights/assistance, 135,136,
    138–141,145
  National Spokesman newsletter, 142
  publications and AV materials, 144
  Training and Placement Service
    (TAPS), 93,123,124,143
Epilepsy School Alert, 83
Epileptologists, 17

Erythromycin, interactions with
  anticonvulsants, 36
Ethosuximide (Zarontin), 32
  in breast milk, 115
Exercise, 70
  sports, 92–93

"Falling sickness," 5
Family
  influences, adult success, 103–104
  role in treatment, 3
  see also Parents
Fear of rejection, 106
Federation for Children with Special
  Needs, 145,147
Fee-for-service health insurance, 127
Fetus
  effects on, 113–114
  origin of seizure disorder, 12,56
Fever, cause of seizures, 58,62,63
First-aid. *See under* Seizure(s)
Food and Drug Administration,
  37,67,157–160
Food stamps, 149
Friends, making, 73–74

General assistance, 148
Generalized epilepsy, 8,9
General physicians, 17,20
Generic anticonvulsants, 37–38
Georgia, comprehensive epilepsy
  program, 143
Godlee, Dr. Rickman J., 41
Grand mal seizure, 9
Grieving process, at learning diagnosis,
  71–72

Half-lives, anticonvulsants, 33
Head injuries, 12
Health care, 15–20,143–144
  changes in provision of, 15–17
  choosing a doctor, 17–19,20
    general physicians, 17,20
    neurologists, 17–20
  costs, 15
  insurance coverage, 18
Health-care team, 4,21–25
  doctor–patient relationship, 23–24
  nurse-clinician role, 24–25
  patient as member, 21–22
  pharmacists, 25
  psychologist, 25
  referrals to other physicians, 24
  social worker, 25
Health insurance, 18,125–129
  state risk pools, 129

Oregon, comprehensive epilepsy
program, 143
Outgrowing epilepsy, 64,87

Parents, of children with epilepsy,
71–74,85,86,100,145,147–152
Partial epilepsy, 8,9
complex cf. simple, 9
Patient
feelings about epilepsy, 3–4
as member of health-care team, 21–22
preparation for surgery, 46–47
PET scans, 28,155–156
Pharmacist, health-care team, 25
Phenobarbital (Luminal), 32
in breast milk, 115
fetal effects, 114
Phenylketonuria (PKU), 11,12
Phenytoin (Dilantin), 32
side-effects, 32,36–37
PKU, 11,12
Preferred provider organization (PPO),
16,128
Pregnancy, 107–108,109–117
anticonvulsants, 37
baby's chances of having epilepsy,
115–116
complications, 114
medication, 110,115,116
birth defects, 107,110–112
breastfeeding, 115,116
effect on baby, 114
planning for, 109, 116–117
seizures during, 112–113
fetus, effect on, 113–114
tonic–clonic, 113
sleep, importance, 112,113,115,116
smoking, avoid, 112,114,117
vitamin K_1 supplementation, 114,117
Primidone (Mysoline), 32
in breast milk, 115
Prison populations, high rates of
epilepsy, 138–139
Professional counseling, adults with
epilepsy, 98,103
Psychogenic seizures, 9–10
Psychologist, health-care team, 25
Publications on epilepsy, 144
Public education, epilepsy, 53
Public transportation/services, legal
issues, 136–137,140

Rebellious behavior, adolescents with
epilepsy, 90–91
Rectal anticonvulsants, childhood
emergencies, 64

Referrals to other physicians, health-care
team, 24
Rehabilitative Services Administration,
123
Rejection, fear of, 106
Research, 153–160
basic science, 153–154
clinical, 158–159
medication, 158–159
developmental, 154–158
animal research, 156,157–158
medication, 156–157
NIH, 154,157–158
supporting, 159–160
Respite care, 80–81,150

Safety
career planning, 119
children, seizures/epilepsy in, 68–69,77
first aid. *See under* Seizure(s)
sports, 92–93
School, children with seizures, 81–83
Seizure(s)
definition, 7–8
EEG, 7,9,10
first aid for, 49–53
children, 77
emergencies, 52
injury prevention, 50,51
medical alert bracelet, 51
put nothing in mouth, 50,51
recognizing seizure, 49–50
status epilepticus, 49,52
tonic–clonic, 49–50,51,52
workplace, 122–123
focus of, determining, for surgical
treatment, 42
newborns and infants, 54–60
during pregnancy, 112–113
threshold, 2–3
treatment, 12; *see also* Anticonvulsant
medication; Surgical treatment
types, 9–10,26,29
see also Epilepsy; *specific aspects*
Seizure diary, 34–36
Seizure disorder cf. epilepsy, 61–62
Self-esteem, 118,124
Self-help groups, 151
Self-image, positive, children, 74–76,83
Sexuality, 105–107
adolescents, 89–90
birth control, 107,109
see also Pregnancy
Sexually transmitted diseases, 107
Siblings, informing, 76–78
Simple partial seizure, 9
Skin rash, anticonvulsants, 34

RC
372
.L58
1990